The Essential Revision Guide to Paediatric Cardiology

REBECCA CASANS

MBBS, MRCPCH
Specialist Registrar in Paediatrics
James Cook University Hospital
South Tees Hospitals NHS Trust, Middlesbrough

MITHILESH LAL

MD, MRCP, FRCPCH
Consultant Paediatrician and Neonatologist
James Cook University Hospital
South Tees Hospitals NHS Trust, Middlesbrough
Examiner, MRCPCH and DCH

and

MICHAEL GRIKSAITIS

MBBS(Hons), MRCPCH, PGDipMedEd
Specialist Registrar in Paediatric Cardiology
Southampton General Hospital
University Hospital Southampton NHS Foundation Trust

Foreword by
DR CHRISTOPHER WREN
MBChB, PhD, FRCP, FRCPCH
Consultant Paediatric Cardiologist
Freeman Hospital, Newcastle upon Tyne

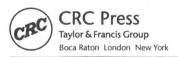

CRC Press
Taylor & Francis Group
Boca Raton London New York

CRC Press is an imprint of the
Taylor & Francis Group, an **informa** business

First published 2013 by Radcliffe Publishing

Published 2021 by CRC Press
Taylor & Francis Group
6000 Broken Sound Parkway NW, Suite 300
Boca Raton, FL 33487-2742

ISBN-13: 978-1-84619-968-4 (pbk)

Contents

Foreword   iv

Preface   v

Acknowledgements   vi

Accreditations   vii

1   Royal College of Paediatrics and Child Health examination structure   1

2   Basic cardiac anatomy, physiology and pharmacology   10

3   Examination of the cardiovascular system   36

4   Interpretation of the paediatric ECG   41

5   Investigations for suspected cardiac disorders   57

6   A–Z of paediatric cardiac disorders and procedures   64

7   Hot topics: a quick reference guide   212
     Ten common problems/diagnoses in paediatric cardiology   213
     Ten common presenting complaints in paediatric cardiology   217

Appendix: reference tables, normal values   219

Glossary   227

Index   233

Foreword

Paediatric cardiology is a subject rich in physical signs and in images produced by investigations (ECGs, X-rays, echocardiograms, angiograms, etc.), making it a compelling and rewarding specialty. It deals mostly with congenital heart defects and arrhythmias, but acquired cardiac problems and cardiac manifestations of more general disease processes are also common.

Cardiovascular malformations affect about 1% of all live born babies, making them as a group the commonest congenital malformations. Advances in diagnosis and treatment have led to an enormous improvement in survival in less than one generation so that almost all babies with previously fatal malformations, such as ventricular septal defect, coarctation of the aorta, tetralogy of Fallot and transposition of the great arteries, are now expected to survive childhood.

Most infants and children with cardiac problems present first to a general paediatrician or neonatologist, often with non-specific symptoms, so familiarity with the history, examination and primary investigations is most important. The aim of this handbook is to provide a rapid and reliable reference to congenital and acquired cardiac problems. It is very well organised with an alphabetical guide to the main diagnoses and investigations as well as a guide to the commonest clinical problems and a differential diagnosis for each mode of presentation. It also provides a more detailed discussion of cardiac physiology and pathophysiology and a comprehensive guide to ECG interpretation. It should be of particular interest to paediatricians in training, including those studying for higher professional examinations, but it also provides a valuable source of reference for paediatricians already in practice.

Dr Christopher Wren
MBChB, PhD, FRCP, FRCPCH
Consultant Paediatric Cardiologist
Freeman Hospital, Newcastle upon Tyne
September 2012

Preface

Continuing on the theme of *The Essential Revision Guide* series in Paediatrics, we are pleased to present this one on *Paediatric Cardiology*. Newborns and children presenting with cardiac conditions is a regular and common occurrence in general paediatric and neonatal units both in district general hospitals and in the specialist regional cardiac centres.

This is a unique reference book; it will take the reader from the relevant basic sciences of cardiac anatomy, physiology and pharmacology through to the initial clinical assessment and investigation of children with known and suspected heart disease. A practical chapter on 'Interpretation of the paediatric ECG' will guide the reader step by step through the analysis of the child's ECG. The layout is distinctive in terms of its general approach, including clinical examination, cardiac investigations followed by an A to Z of specific conditions and procedures in alphabetical order. The book concludes with '10 hot topics' and a list of key differential diagnoses associated with common presentations. An appendix containing blood pressure centile tables, ECG reference ranges and basic cardiac catheter data completes the book.

This book is primarily intended for all healthcare professionals involved in the care of children at the point of presentation. It will be of particular relevance to paediatricians in training, general practitioners, emergency department staff and specialist nurses. It will also provide a useful reference guide for those staff working in specialist regional cardiac centres.

The content of this book will meet the requirements of the core curricula for paediatricians in training at all levels. Those taking either the written or clinical components of the MRCPCH exam will find this book an essential tool. All candidates taking the part 2 clinical examination will be assessed on a clinical aspect of paediatric cardiology. Candidates sitting the Diploma in Child Health (DCH) examination will also benefit greatly from this book. Those taking postgraduate examinations in other specialties involved in the care of children will also find this a useful reference guide.

As always we will strongly rely on the feedback from readers to make significant revisions and further improvements in future editions.

Rebecca Casans
Mithilesh Lal
Michael Griksaitis
September 2012

Acknowledgements

We are grateful for the endless hours of cardiology teaching provided by Dr Christopher Wren and his ongoing support in the writing of this book.

We would like to thank Dr Shankar Sadagopan for his critical review of this book.

Finally, we would like to thank all of our families for their ongoing support!

Accreditations

The following figures have been adapted with permission from original sources:

Figure 2.9

Frontiers in Bioscience
- Catalucci D *et al*. Physiological myocardial hypertrophy: how and why. *Frontiers in Bioscience*. 2008; 13: 312–24.

Figure 2.10

Oxford University Press
- Holte K *et al*. Pathophysiology and clinical implications of perioperative fluid excess. *British Journal of Anaesthesia*. 2002; 89(4): 622–32.

Figure 2.11

Elsevier
- Jain KS, Bariwal JB, Kathiravan MK *et al*. Recent advances in selective α1-adrenoreceptor antagonists as antihypertensive agents. *Bioorganic & Medicinal Chemistry*. 2008; 16(9): 4759–800.

Figures 6.22, 6.46

Richard Kirk, www.crkirk.com

Figures 6.4, 6.24, 6.36, 6.51, 6.52, 6.59A, 6.59C

Radiological Society of North America
- Gaca AM, Jaggers JJ, Dudley LT *et al*. Repair of congenital heart disease: a primer – part 1. *Radiology*. 2008; **247**: 617–31.
- Gaca AM, Jaggers JJ, Dudley LT *et al*. Repair of congenital heart disease: a primer – part 2. *Radiology*. 2008; **248**: 44–60.

Figure 6.30

Future Science Group
- Matsui H, Adachi I, Uemura H *et al*. Anatomy of coarctation, hypoplastic and interrupted aortic arch: relevance to interventional/surgical treatment. *Expert Review of Cardiovascular Therapy*. 2007; 5(5): 871–80.

Figure 6.34

Reproduced with permission and copyright of Tufts University.

Blood pressure levels for boys and girls

National Heart, Lung, and Blood Institute (NHLBI)

RC: To Fida with love.
ML: Dedicated to my wife Anita
MG: Dedicated to my parents, Mary and Peter
and brothers, David and Christopher.

Royal College of Paediatrics and Child Health examination structure

Part 1 A and B written
Part 2 written
Part 2 clinical examination

RCPCH: EXAMINATION STRUCTURE

This chapter aims to explain the process of paediatric assessment set out by the Royal College of Paediatrics and Child Health (RCPCH). It will be useful to new paediatric trainees in preparation for membership examination and for non-trainees to gain an insight into the college examination process.

The RCPCH has a robust assessment strategy and it is set in the context of paediatric training. The assessment process itself is transparent and uses a range of different assessment methods, including written examinations to test theory and a practical examination to assess practical skills.

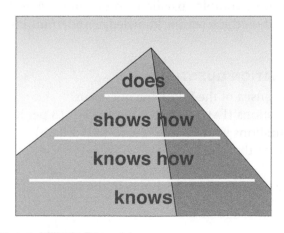

does	Workplace
shows how	Clinical Examination
knows how	Applied Test
knows	MCQ Examination

FIGURE 1.1 Miller's Pyramid

This concept is nicely demonstrated by Miller's Pyramid which maps different methods of assessment.

Note: All of the following information has been taken from the RCPCH website with permission and is correct at time of publication, though subject to change. Please see the website www.rcpch.co.uk for further details.

THE INDIVIDUAL PARTS OF MRCPCH

Part 1A

This is a single written paper which aims to test basic clinical knowledge in paediatrics. Trainees should be able to pass this paper having completed at least 4 months of clinical paediatrics and after engagement in self-directed learning from any good, short paediatric textbook. This has a pass rate of 60%–70% among UK trainees.

Part 1A is also taken in the UK by trainees wishing to complete the Diploma in Child Health. This assessment is aimed at those intending a career, including the care of children, but not where this is the main component of their daily work. It is principally taken by general practitioners.

Part 1B

This is a single written paper. It aims principally to test the understanding and science which underpins paediatric practice. This has a pass rate of 25%–30% among UK trainees. Currently, this low pass rate is a matter of concern which is being specifically addressed.

➤ **Paper 1a** focuses on the areas of child health that are relevant to those who will be working with children in their medical careers, not just those entering mainstream hospital-based paediatrics. The areas to be tested will be those conditions likely to be seen in 6 to 12 months of hospital, community or primary care practice. This paper also serves as the written component of the Diploma in Child Health examination.

➤ **Paper 1b** focuses on the more complex paediatric problem-solving skills not tested in Paper 1a, and on the scientific knowledge underpinning paediatrics.

THE NUMBER OF EXAMINATION QUESTIONS

Paper 1a and Paper 1b will consist of the following questions:
➤ 2 extended matching questions (EMQ) worth 9 marks each (3 per item)
➤ 15 multiple true-false questions worth 5 marks each (1 per item)
➤ 48 best of five questions worth 4 marks each

Both Paper 1a and Paper 1b papers will be 2½ hours in duration.

QUESTION TYPES

Multiple true-false questions

Multiple true-false questions are most useful when testing knowledge when there is an absolute Yes/No answer.

The questions test whether a candidate has true knowledge of a fact or thinks that something similar (but wrong) sounds vaguely familiar.

A simple statement or short clinical scenario leads into five items, e.g.

➤ 'The following statements about X condition are true:'
➤ 'X is a complication of'.

Alternatively, they might test whether a candidate has true knowledge of a fact or thinks that something similar (but wrong) sounds vaguely familiar, e.g.

➤ 'Characteristic features of X condition include'

Best of Five questions

Best of Five questions are used to test judgement and experience. A simple statement or short clinical scenario leads into five options. All could be possible, but only one is completely correct or more correct than the others.

They should cover only one aspect of the topic, so stems might be:

➤ 'What is the most likely diagnosis?'
➤ 'Which investigation is most likely to lead to a diagnosis?'
➤ 'What is the best next step?'
➤ 'What is the best advice to give to parents?'
➤ 'What is the most likely pathogenesis of this condition?'
➤ 'What is the most common cause of this?'

Extended matching questions

Extended matching questions are used in much the same way as Best of Five questions. In this case a list of 10 possible answers is offered with three statements or clinical scenarios.

The candidate chooses the best option from the introductory list. Again, all could be possible, but only one is completely correct or more correct than the others.

EMQs are often accompanied by laboratory results that are similar but with differences. They should cover only one aspect of the topic, so suitable questions might be as follows.

➤ 'Choose the most likely diagnosis from the following:'
➤ 'Choose the best treatment for each of these children:'
➤ 'Choose the organism which matches most closely each of the following case scenarios:'

PART 2 WRITTEN

This is an applied knowledge test. It comprises a single examination divided into two papers over a day. Most of the questions are based on clinical scenarios. A child is described, for example, who is admitted with certain symptoms. The findings on examination are given. This is often followed or accompanied by X-rays, investigations or laboratory results.

The candidate is asked to select the most likely diagnosis or the most important steps in management. Other questions may address therapeutics, follow-up or referral to colleagues. Success in this examination demands knowledge and clinical training with experience. This examination has a pass rate of 40%–50% among UK trainees.

The MRCPCH Part 2 consists of two papers, each of 2½ hours' duration.

The examination is a test of clinical knowledge and decision making in all areas of paediatrics and child health. The two-paper format offers the opportunity to examine widely across the curriculum and to improve coverage of all major areas of clinical practice, so the validity of the examination will be increased. This format allows the MRCPCH Part 2 Board to include questions in the papers dealing with research, audit, ethics and medical science applied to clinical care. Some material on adolescent medicine will be included in the examination.

➤ Each paper will carry approximately the same number of marks.
➤ Candidate's marks will be combined from the two papers to form an overall mark.
➤ The standard of the examination is still set at the level of knowledge expected of a competent paediatrician in training entering into core higher specialist training.
➤ Each paper will consist of a mixture of questions which are known as case histories, data interpretation, and photographic material.
➤ The questions set will be a combination of new format questions and will include 'best of' list, 'n from many' list and 'extended matching' questions.

Question format

Photographic material

Each question is based upon printed photographic material. The photographs are prepared from clinical and retinal photographs, radiographs, illustrations of investigation results and occasionally from pathological material. Candidates are asked to identify abnormalities, or provide a diagnosis, to recommend investigation or treatment or a combination of these.

Case history

Each question will be a case history with results of physical examination and investigations. The questions are designed to test ability in diagnosis and in the planning of investigations and management, and they may be extended to include photographic material.

Data interpretation

Each question will consist of such items as sets of laboratory data or graphical data; for example, electrocardiograms introduced by a short statement of the clinical setting. Candidates are asked for specific points of interpretation.

Please note that drugs will almost invariably be referred to by their UK approved names rather than their trade names. Biochemical and other measurements will be expressed in SI units (normal ranges or reference ranges will be provided only where these are likely to be in doubt).

Question structure

'Best of' list questions

There is one best answer from a given list. Although all the answers given may be reasonable, one will be the best answer. Marks will be awarded only for choosing the correct answer.

'N from many' questions

A stated number of answers are required from a longer list, e.g. a list of possible diagnoses from an ECG. The candidate is not expected to go through all the options, but to select the answer from the list provided; for example, if the ECG shows complete heart block, find this option in the list.

Extended matching questions

This format employs a list of answers or options. The list is followed by a set of questions or statements. The candidate is required to select, from the list of options, the best match for each of the questions or statements. An example might be a list of causes of wheezing, which need to be matched with the most appropriate of one or more case histories.

Each question on the MRCPCH Part 2 examination carries its own weighting. You will see on the exam paper how many points each question is worth. The maximum score per question will be split by the number of correct responses required. Incorrect responses will gain a score of zero.

PART 2 CLINICAL

The aim of the examination is to assess whether candidates have reached the standard in clinical skills expected of a **newly appointed Specialist Registrar**.

Candidates are expected to demonstrate proficiency in:

➤ communication
➤ history-taking and management planning
➤ establishing rapport with both parents and children
➤ physical examination
➤ child development
➤ clinical judgement
➤ organisation of thoughts and actions

➤ recognition of acute illness
➤ knowledge of paediatrics and child health
➤ professional behaviour
➤ ethical practice.

The MRCPCH Clinical examination follows an OSCE style format. Stations are set to test candidates in:
➤ child development
➤ communication skills
➤ history-taking and management planning
➤ recognition and diagnosis of clinical signs and symptoms
➤ physical examination skills.

NEW MRCPCH CLINICAL EXAMINATION CIRCUIT (Revised January 2009)

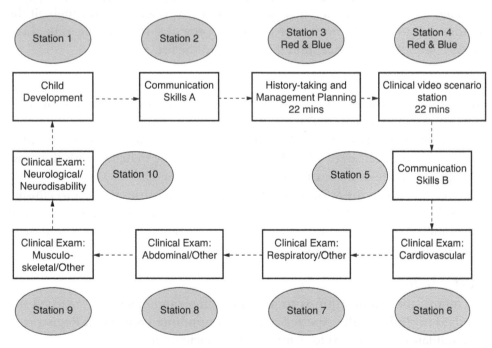

All stations of 9 minutes' duration, except Stations 3 and 4 which are each 22 minutes in length

RCPCH MRCPCH Clinical Examination Cardiovascular mark scheme

Royal College of Paediatrics and Child Health MRCPCH Examination	Clinical Examination Station–CVS	Date:	Time:	Age of child:
		Occasion used (1st, 2nd etc):		

CANDIDATE NUMBER	CANDIDATE NAME	EXAMINER NUMBER		

Please enter candidate number in the grid to the left and print name below

EXAMINER NAME

Please enter examiner number in the grid to the right and print name below

Do not write in this shaded area

Degree of co-operation of child

Compliant ☐
Hesitant ☐
Unwilling ☐

FOR FEEDBACK PURPOSES MARK THE PERFORMANCE IN EACH SECTION   Station 6

Case reference	Special circumstances	

Conduct of Examination	Please mark here →	Clear Pass	Pass	Bare Fail	Clear Fail	Un-acceptable
Rapport, putting child at ease Appropriate confidence and pace Communication with the child		☐	☐	☐	☐	☐

Clinical Examination	Please mark here →	Clear Pass	Pass	Bare Fail	Clear Fail	Un-acceptable
Structured, fluid technique Identification, interpretation of clinical signs Appropriate confidence in clinical findings Demonstration of signs when asked		☐	☐	☐	☐	☐

Discussion with Examiner	Please mark here →	Clear Pass	Pass	Bare Fail	Clear Fail	Un-acceptable
Differential diagnosis. investigation selection Management planning Implications for child and family		☐	☐	☐	☐	☐

Please record your overall judgement of the candidate's performance	MARK FINAL GRADE HERE ▶	Clear Pass	Pass	Bare Fail	Clear Fail	Un-acceptable
		☐	☐	☐	☐	☐

STANDARDS FOR ASSESSMENT: CLINICAL EXAMINATION STATION

RCPCH Anchor Statements

Conduct of examination	**Conduct of examination**
	an understanding of the roles and responsibilities of paediatricians
	effective responses to challenge, complexity and stress in paediatrics
	effective skills in three-way consultation and examination
	an understanding of effective communication and interpersonal skills with children of all ages
	empathy and sensitivity and skills in engaging the trust and consent from children and their families
	an understanding of equality and diversity in paediatric practice
	ethical personal and professional practice
Clinical examination	
	effective skills in paediatric assessment
Discussion with examiners	
	skills in formulating an appropriate differential diagnosis in paediatrics
	effective initial management of ill-health and clinical conditions in paediatrics seeking additional advice and opinion as appropriate *(as outlined in the Framework of Competences for Level 1 in Paediatrics)*
	knowledge of the science-base for paediatrics *(as outlined in the Framework of Competences for Level 1 in Paediatrics)*
	knowledge of common and serious paediatric conditions and their management
	an understanding of growth, development, health and well-being in paediatrics

Please turn over for more detailed advice on how to interpret if a candidate has reached these standards

The final mark for each statement is based upon the expert assessment of each candidate's performance, clinical ability and knowledge. These Anchor statements provide a list of the components which contribute to judging a candidate's performance. The importance or relevance of the individual component will vary from station to station.

ANCHOR STATEMENTS: CLINICAL EXAMINATION STATION

Expected standard:	CLEAR PASS	PASS	BARE FAIL	CLEAR FAIL	UNACCEPTABLE
Conduct of examination	Full greetings and introduction. Appropriate level of confidence. Appropriate pace without push. Putting parent/child at ease. Talks and explains examination to child when appropriate. Manner and language adjusted to suit the child	Adequate approach. A little slow or rushed. Child relaxed but not always engaged. Instructions appropriate for child. No major points of poor communication or approach.	Incomplete greeting and introduction. Inadequate identification of aims and objectives. Does not show appropriate level of confidence, empathetic nature or putting parent/child at ease. Failure to engage appropriately with child.	Approach not satisfactory in important area or on frequent occasions. Poor explanation to child of examination. Instructions to child poor. Does not engage child.	Dismissive of parent/child. Lack of civility or politeness. Rudeness or arrogance. Inappropriate manner including flippancy. No communication with child. No explanation of examination.
Clinical examination	Well-structured and systematic examination. Fluent technique. Correctly identifies and interprets clinical signs. Knows whether signs found can be relied upon, and if not why. Displays overall clinical competence.	Majority of clinical skills demonstrated accurately eliciting the majority of physical signs correctly. May need some prompting and may be some lack of fluency.	Misses an important sign or its interpretation but the rest is accurate. Too many minor errors. Examination technique not well structured. Poor fluency of approach.	Misses several important clinical signs or incorrect interpretation. Slow, uncertain unstructured unsystematic examination. Describes non-existent findings.	**Behavioural:** Rough handling of child. Disregards child's distress or shyness or modesty. Describes non-existent findings confidently. **Medical Knowledge/ Competence:** No apparent system or skill in clinical examination. Worryingly incompetent.
Discussion with examiners	Correct differential diagnosis. Suggests appropriate investigation and management. Able to suggest appropriate steps if examination incomplete or inconclusive. Understands implications of findings for child and family.	Correct diagnosis and reasonable discussion of differential and investigations. Main management issues dealt with. Main implications of findings covered.	Incorrect diagnosis or important errors in discussion of diagnosis and differential. Unable to discuss important aspects of management. Inappropriate confidence.	Errors suggest poor understanding or lack of knowledge with significant clinical implications. Confident and wrong.	**Behavioural:** Unable to discuss findings. Dismissive of discussion. Potentially dangerous interpretation. **Medical Knowledge/ Competence:** Level of knowledge that questions medical qualification. Ignorant of important basic knowledge.

The final mark for each statement is based upon the expert assessment of each candidate's performance, clinical ability and knowledge. These Anchor statements provide a list of the components which contribute to judging a candidate's performance. The importance or relevance of the individual component will vary from station to station.

CHAPTER 2

Basic cardiac anatomy, physiology and pharmacology

Basic cardiac anatomy
Introduction
The heart *in situ*
The isolated heart
Anatomy of the cardiac conduction system
The fetal circulation

Basic cardiac physiology
Introduction
The cardiac cycle
Cardiac output
Cardiac function
Cardiac conduction
Control of heart rate
Control of blood pressure
Common receptor sites and their actions

Basic cardiovascular pharmacology
Classification of drugs groups
A to Z of common drugs

BASIC CARDIAC ANATOMY

Introduction

Before embarking on studying paediatric cardiology, it is important to have a basic understanding of cardiac anatomy, as the majority of this specialty is based around congenital heart disease. To appreciate the abnormal heart, you need to understand what the normal anatomy is.

This section reviews the relevant gross cardiac and vascular anatomy relevant to paediatricians. It also includes short descriptions of the anatomy of the electrical conduction system and fetal circulation.

The heart *in situ*

The heart is a muscular structure, just larger than the clenched fist of the individual. It sits within the middle division of the mediastinum. The heart is rotated within the chest so that when facing a patient, the anterior surface of the heart is predominantly composed of the right atria and right ventricle. The left atria and left ventricle are therefore posterior. This concept is important when considering placement of ECG leads (e.g. V1–3 will look at the anterior surface of the heart – hence look at the right ventricle) or the palpation of heaves during clinical examination. The orientation of the heart within the chest is displayed in Figure 2.1 below.

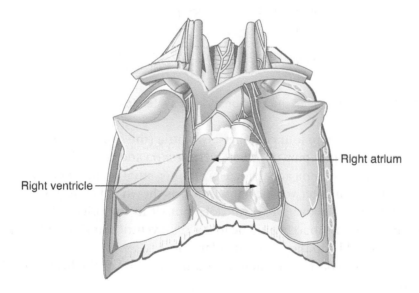

FIGURE 2.1 Anterior chest wall dissected to show that the right atrium and right ventricle are the anterior structures

The heart is contained within the pericardium (a double-walled fibrous structure). The pericardium has several roles including preventing rapid overfilling of the heart and allowing the heart to beat in a frictionless environment. There is a tiny serous-filled space between the two layers of the pericardium, known as the pericardial space. This space has the potential to expand and fill with fluid in certain conditions, or in trauma to the chest. The pericardium is susceptible to disease processes including pericarditis and pericardial effusions, which are discussed later in this book.

The isolated heart

The heart is split into two sides: a right side dealing with deoxygenated blood returning from the systemic circulation then going to the lungs, and a left side dealing with oxygenated blood returning from the lungs and then going around the body. These circulations should not mix in normal health. This concept is displayed in Figure 2.2.

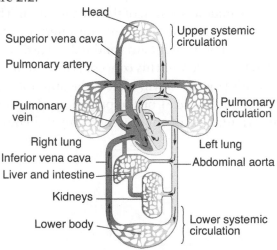

FIGURE 2.2 Interactions of the pulmonary and systemic circulations

The heart is made of up four chambers: two atria (the collecting chambers) and two ventricles (the pumping chambers). These atria and ventricles are divided by tissue valves. The two atria are divided by an inter-atrial septum and the two ventricles divided by an inter-ventricular septum, as shown in Figure 2.3. Remember that, as mentioned above, the heart does not sit in the orientation as shown below. The anterior surface would be to the right ventricular side and the posterior surface would be to the left ventricular side.

Important concepts to remember regarding anatomy of the heart include the following.

➤ The apex of the heart should point to the left side of the chest.

➤ There should be one superior vena cava (SVC) returning to the right atria. However, a small number of the population (especially those with congenital heart disease) can have an additional 'left SVC'. This is not usually a problem; the left SVC usually drains into the coronary sinus, which then drains into the right atria (hence no mixing of oxygenated or deoxygenated blood).

➤ Four pulmonary veins return from the lungs to the left atria (two from the right lung and two from the left lung). It is possible to have all of these veins draining elsewhere (known as total anomalous pulmonary venous drainage) or some returning to the left atrium and the remainder elsewhere (known as partial anomalous pulmonary venous drainage).

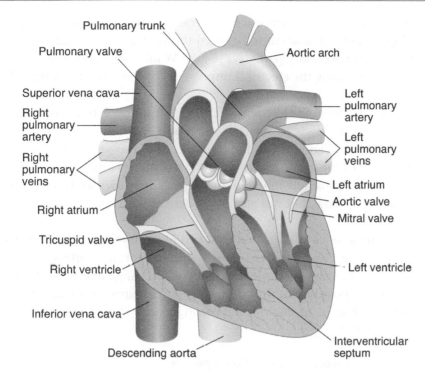

FIGURE 2.3 Interior structure of the heart and great vessels

➤ Both the atrial and ventricular septa should prevent blood flow between each side of the heart. The exception is in the fetus (see below) and in the initial newborn period where the foramen ovale may still be open for a short while. Defects in either the atrial or ventricular septum are known as an atrial septal defect (ASD) or ventricular septal defect (VSD), and a defect in both the atrial and ventricular septa is known as an atrioventricular septal defect (AVSD).

➤ The inter-ventricular septum is mostly a muscular structure, although the very top of the septum is known as the 'perimembranous' region and does not contain muscle. This is important when classifying ventricular septal defects and predicting their natural history.

➤ The left ventricle (LV) is the usual dominant ventricle after the neonatal period, and should form the apex of the heart. Although the LV has a slightly thicker muscular wall, both the LV and the right ventricle (RV) should be similar in size (a well-balanced heart). Major discrepancy in ventricular size leads you to consider a major structural heart defect (e.g. hypoplastic left heart syndrome, tricuspid atresia).

➤ The tricuspid valve is slightly lower than the mitral valve. This is known as an 'offset' of the valves. This offset is lost in complete atrioventricular septal defects, and is enhanced in Ebstein's anomaly, with a very low set tricuspid valve.

➤ The ring of fibrous tissue around the mitral and tricuspid valves is important in acting as electrical insulation between the atria and the ventricles. This is often the site of accessory pathways (e.g. in Wolff–Parkinson–White (WPW) syndrome), allowing the electrical impulse to 'bypass' the atrioventricular node.

➤ The aorta arises from the left ventricle. The pulmonary artery arises from the right ventricle. These two vessels 'cross over' each other as they exit (demonstrated in Figure 2.3). This crossover of the vessels is lost in transposition of the great arteries, where both arteries arise in parallel.

➤ The aortic valve is usually made up of three leaflets (tricuspid). Bicuspid valves can be normal, but can also be associated with coarctation of the aorta.

➤ The coronary arteries arise from the ascending aorta, shortly after it exits the left ventricle. Usually, there is a right and left coronary artery, although variations exist between people, especially when congenital heart disease is present. It is possible for the coronary arteries to arise from abnormal locations, such as in anomalous left coronary artery from the pulmonary artery (ALCAPA).

Anatomy of the cardiac conduction system

The heart has its own intrinsic pacemaker system, although this can be affected by extrinsic factors such as catecholamines (e.g. adrenaline).

The first pacemaker is known as the sinoatrial node (SAN). The SAN is a collection of specialised cells that have the ability to initiate short bursts of electrical impulses. The SAN is located in the right atrium, at the junction of the SVC to the right atrium (RA). The SAN's role is to initiate the electrical activity that will ultimately result in a 'heartbeat' after its journey through the conduction system.

Specialised bundles of conduction tissue exist within the atria, allowing the impulses from the SAN to travel throughout the atria, causing depolarisation.

The impulses then arrive at the second of the heart's pacemakers, the atrioventricular node (AVN). The AVN is a smaller collection of cells than the SAN and is located at the lower part of the inter-atrial septum, at the opening of the coronary sinus into the RA.

The impulse passes through the AVN (following a short time delay) and down the bundle of His; this is a group of fibres that act as a bridge between the myocardium of the atrium and the ventricles. It should be the only anatomical site that electrical impulses can cross through the fibrous insulating layer of the mitral and tricuspid valves.

At the top of the muscular aspect of the inter-ventricular septum the bundle of His divides into the right and left bundles, also known as fascicles (the left bundle then goes on to divide into a left anterior and posterior bundle). These bundles pass around the ventricular myocardium, producing small branches known as Purkinje fibres, to transmit the electrical impulse.

The impulse terminates as it migrates up the walls of the LV and RV and meets the insulating layer of tissue once again. Any surgery within the heart has the risk of damaging any part of the conduction system, giving the risk of post-operative heart blocks, bundle branch blocks or arrhythmias.

The anatomy of the electrical conduction system is demonstrated in Figure 2.4.

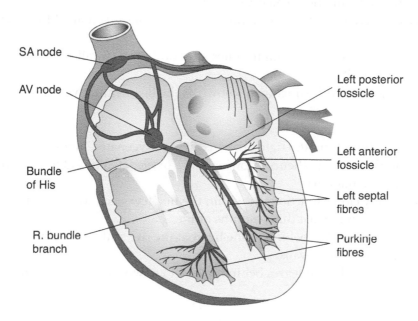

FIGURE 2.4 Anatomy of the cardiac electrical conduction system

The fetal circulation

Special mention needs to be given to the anatomy of the fetal circulation, given the role of paediatricians caring for preterm infants and term newborns. The fetal circulation has an overall structure similar to that described above. However, there are some differences that can cause clinical problems after birth.

The fetus has very high pulmonary vascular resistance (due to amniotic fluid in the developing lung and vasoconstricted pulmonary vasculature). This means that the right ventricle is under higher pressure than the left ventricle and so the RV becomes the dominant ventricle. The right-sided pressures are higher in a fetus than the left side. Persistence of these high right-sided pressures in newborn life causes a problem known as persistent pulmonary hypertension of the newborn (PPHN).

Secondly, the fetus does not need to deliver blood flow to the lung parenchyma; the oxygenation of the blood is provided by the mother. The fetus can also deal very well with hypoxia. As a result, three shunts are present in the fetus that help to redirect the majority of oxygenated blood around the systemic circulation and bypass the lungs (although please note that some blood does go to the lung to provide oxygen to enable the fetal lung tissue to develop). These shunts (in the order encountered by the blood leaving the mother and entering fetus) are as follows.

1 Ductus venosus
➤ This joins the umbilical vein (carrying oxygenated blood from mother) directly to the inferior vena cava (IVC).
➤ It is a bypass through the liver, preventing a lot of oxygenated blood being consumed by the liver.
➤ It closes functionally within minutes after birth. Structurally closes within first week of life.
➤ The remnant of this structure is known as the ligamentum venosum.

2 Foramen ovale
➤ This is a shunt from the right atria (receiving oxygenated blood from the IVC) to the left atria (hence allowing more oxygenated blood to enter the systemic circulation).
➤ It normally closes functionally within the first few weeks of life and structurally in the first three months of life.
➤ The indentation left behind in the heart at the site of the foramen ovale is known as the fossa ovalis.
➤ If it does not close, it leaves behind a defect known as a patent foramen ovale (PFO).

3 Ductus arteriosus
➤ This is a shunt between the pulmonary artery and the aorta, allowing any blood in the pulmonary artery (under high pressure in a fetus) to be diverted to the systemic system via the aorta (under low pressure in a fetus).
➤ The ductus arteriosus closes quickly after birth in a term infant, although some flow can be detected for up to a week or more in some children with no consequence.
➤ If the ductus arteriosus persists it becomes known as a patent ductus arteriosus (PDA), which can have haemodynamic consequences (*see* page 150)
➤ The remnant of this structure when closed is known as the ligamentum arteriosum.

The anatomy of the fetal circulation is displayed in Figure 2.5.
   Many changes occur immediately after birth when the neonate takes its first breath and begins to aerate its lungs:
1   Increase in PaO2
2   Fall in pulmonary vascular resistance
3   Rise in systemic vascular resistance
4   Decrease in heart rate (a fetus has a higher heart rate)

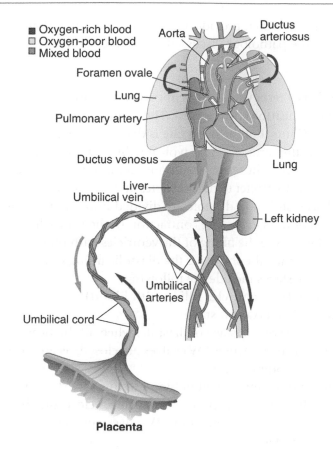

■ Oxygen-rich blood
□ Oxygen-poor blood
▨ Mixed blood

Aorta

Ductus arteriosus

Foramen ovale

Lung

Pulmonary artery

Ductus venosus

Lung

Liver
Umbilical vein

Left kidney

Umbilical arteries

Umbilical cord

Placenta

FIGURE 2.5 Anatomy of the fetal circulation

5 Closure of all three shunts begins
6 Any shunt that remains open should gradually change from being a right to left shunt to bi-directional shunt to ultimately left to right.

Many of these changes have clinically noticeable effects in clinical examination, pathological signs in heart disease and on investigation findings (such as electrocardiogram (ECG)).

Summary

It is important to have a basic understanding of anatomy to help understand the congenital defects, arrhythmias and neonatal heart disease. Having this understanding will also make explaining defects to parents easier for you and them!

BASIC CARDIOVASCULAR PHYSIOLOGY

Introduction

This section aims to identify key areas of physiology that are important to paediatricians caring for children with heart disease. It is not a comprehensive textbook discussion. It will, however, provide a good understanding that you can subsequently apply to the pathology discussed in this textbook.

The cardiac cycle

The cardiac cycle is a term used to describe the events that take place within the heart between one heartbeat to the next. The heart rate determines the speed of the cardiac cycle. Control of the heart rate is discussed separately below.

On a basic level the cardiac cycle is typically divided into a systolic period and a diastolic period. When the terms systole and diastole are used in general day-to-day clinical practice, they refer to the ventricles and *not* the atria. This is important to understand, as systole and diastole are divided into different parts. The ventricular systolic period relates to the contraction of the ventricles; the ventricular diastolic period relates to the filling of the ventricles with blood (*see* Figure 2.6). The faster the heart rate, the shorter is the diastolic filling time.

The cardiac cycle stages include the following.

1 **Diastolic phase (i.e. ventricles filling with blood)**
   a. **Isovolumetric relaxation stage**
      ➤ This is the very first stage of diastole, when all the heart is relaxed and the atrioventricular (AV) valves are closed, as are the outlet valves (aortic and pulmonary).
      ➤ There is no net movement of blood in this very short initial stage.
      ➤ It starts from the moment the outlet valves close and the cessation of systole. It ends the moment the AV valves open and the blood starts to pass through.
   b. **Rapid filling**
      ➤ This is the second stage of the diastolic phase.
      ➤ In this stage the ventricles are under lower pressure than the atria, and so blood passively moves from the atria into the ventricles.
      ➤ This stage accounts for most of the ventricular filling.
      ➤ It starts from the moment that blood crosses the AV valves and ends when the atrial and ventricular pressures are equal (i.e. no gradient between the two chambers).
   c. **Diastasis**
      ➤ This is the third stage of the diastolic phase when the atria and ventricles are at equal pressure.
      ➤ As a result, no blood moves through the AV valves in this stage.
      ➤ It usually occurs in mid-diastole.
   d. **Atrial systole**
      ➤ This is the final stage of the diastolic phase.
      ➤ The atria contract, generating a sudden pressure that exceeds the ventricular pressure and a second wave of blood flow through the AV valve into the ventricles.

➤ This stage is important for emptying the final blood volume within the atria.

➤ The atrial contraction accounts for 10%–20% of the total cardiac output due to atrial systole (hence when in an atrial arrhythmia with reduced atrial function, the cardiac output will fall if this stage is affected).

2 **Systolic phase** (i.e. ventricular contraction to generate blood flow around body)

   a. **Isovolumetric contraction**

   ➤ This is the first stage of systole.

   ➤ It occurs when the ventricles start to contract, raising the intra-ventricular pressure, causing the AV valves to close, preventing regurgitation of blood through the AV valves back into the atria.

   ➤ However, the ventricles are still initially under lower pressure than the outlet vessels and so there is no net movement of blood.

   ➤ This stage ends as soon as the outlet valves (aortic and pulmonary) open.

   b. **Ejection**

   ➤ This stage is responsible for the emptying of the ventricles into the outlet vessels to allow the delivery of blood to the pulmonary and systemic circulations.

   ➤ It starts as soon as the outlet valves open and the ventricular pressure exceeds the outlet vessel pressure.

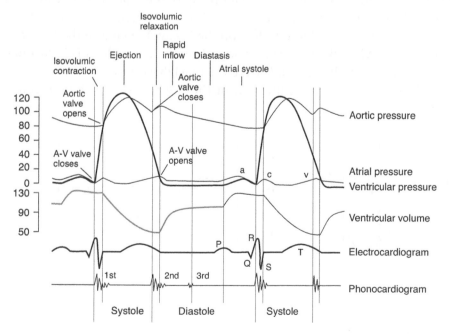

FIGURE 2.6 The events during the cardiac cycle

➤ Once the ventricular pressure has fallen as they empty their contents, the outlet valves close to prevent regurgitation of blood back into the ventricles and the cardiac cycle starts again with isovolumetric relaxation (stage one of diastole).

Figure 2.6 provides a graphical summary of the events during the cardiac cycle. It clearly demonstrates how the atrial and ventricular pressures change, and as a result changes the volume of blood in these chambers.

Pay close attention in Figure 2.7 to the relationship of the phases of the cardiac cycle to the heart sounds and the ECG. These are two useful points to remember regarding the cardiac cycle for use in day-to-day clinical work.

The first heart sound (HS1) you hear (caused by the closure of the AV valves) signifies the start of systole. The second heart sound (HS2) you hear (caused by the closure of the outlet valves) signifies the end of systole, or in fact the start of diastole (Figure 2.7). You can use this concept to help with the assessment of murmurs (*see* Chapter 3, page 39).

HS1 ⟷ HS2 ⟷ HS1 ⟷ HS2 ⟷ HS1

Systole   *Diastole*   *Systole*   *Diastole*

FIGURE 2.7 Relationship of the heart sounds (HS) to the periods in the cardiac cycle

The final point to remember is the relationship of the phases of the cardiac cycle to the ECG. The (ventricular) systolic period often referred to corresponds to the start of the peak of the QRS complex (on the R wave). It ends at the termination of the T wave. While the P wave corresponds to atrial systole, it is in fact part of the ventricular diastolic period. The (ventricular) diastolic period corresponds to the end of the T wave, until the start of the R wave. This is demonstrated in Figure 2.8.

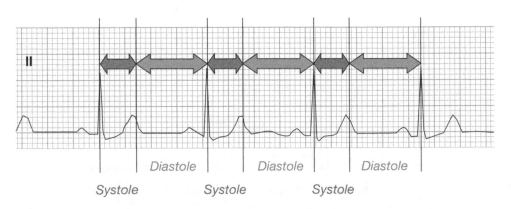

FIGURE 2.8 Relationship of the ECG waves to the periods in the cardiac cycle

Cardiac output

The role of the heart is to generate a cardiac output (volume of blood pumped out of one ventricle in one minute) to the pulmonary circulation (from the right ventricle) and the systemic circulation (from the left ventricle). You can assess cardiac output clinically (with perfusion, heart rate, blood pressure, pulse volumes, temperature) or using echocardiography or with more invasive monitoring techniques in the Paediatric Intensive Care Unit (PICU). Assessments of cardiac output form a vital part of the assessment of any unwell child (e.g. with meningococcal sepsis, heart failure, trauma etc.). By understanding more about cardiac function and cardiac output you will be in a better position to manage these children.

Cardiac output (CO) can be calculated using the formula:

$$CO = \textit{Stroke Volume (litres/beat)} \times \textit{Heart Rate (beats/minute)}$$

(Stroke volume (SV) is the volume of blood from one ventricle per beat).

Factors determining the cardiac output include the following.
➤ **Cardiac function** (i.e. the ability for the heart to contract; see below)
  ➢ If the cardiac function is poor, the CO will be low.
  ➢ It is also important that atrial function is good to ensure the ventricles are well filled.
➤ **Heart rate**
  ➢ To a certain point, increasing your heart rate will increase your CO.
  ➢ However, if too tachycardic (e.g. with supraventricular tachycardia (SVT)) the diastolic filling period is too short, and so CO will fall.
➤ **Ventricular preload** (the volume of blood returning to the heart and filling the ventricle)
  ➢ Increasing venous return to the heart will increase the ventricular end diastolic pressure and increase myocardial stretching, which in turn will increase the SV.
  ➢ However, if too much fluid is given and the heart is overstretched the contractility and then SV will fall (Starling's Law of the Heart), so a balance needs to be reached.
➤ **Ventricular afterload** (the pressure the ventricles must overcome to eject blood)
  ➢ The higher the afterload the lower the CO, as the ventricle will have a greater residual volume at the end of the contraction.

Cardiac function

Cardiac function is important to ensure good CO, and hence oxygen delivery to tissues. A normal functional heart requires:
➤ a structurally normal heart (i.e. no major congenital heart disease)

➤ normal myocardium (i.e. no metabolic or muscular diseases)
➤ an oxygen supply to the myocardium (i.e. normal coronary perfusion)
➤ a suitable preload (i.e. normal venous return to the heart)
➤ a suitable afterload (i.e. a suitable systemic blood pressure).

We can assess cardiac function by making direct or indirect assessments of the CO or by assessing the contractility of the myocardium. Contractility is defined as the force of contraction for a given fibre length within the myocardium.

Contractility is explained by Starling's Law of the Heart. This states that 'the energy released during contraction depends upon the initial fibre length'. This means that the greater the heart is stretched by ventricular filling, the energy (and so force) of the contraction will be greater (Figure 2.9). This works until a certain ventricular volume, after which the heart becomes overstretched (with less actin-myosin connections in the cardiac muscle), which results in a reduced contractility and a consequential decrease in cardiac output (Figure 2.10). The significance of this is high; many children do need fluid resuscitation, but do not give them excessive fluid. This is particularly important in neonates.

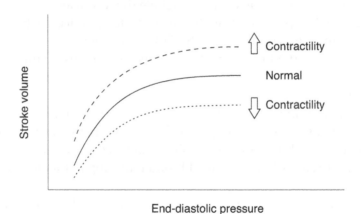

FIGURE 2.9 Curve illustrating Starling's law, demonstrating positive and negative inotropic lines

The term positive inotropic effect is used to describe moving from the normal line to the increased contractility (therefore an increased CO at the same end-diastolic volume). Causes of positive inotropic effects include:
➤ inotropic drugs (e.g. dopamine, dobutamine, adrenaline, noradrenaline)
➤ exercise
➤ increased temperature.

The term negative inotropic effect is used to describe moving down from the normal line to the reduced contractility (therefore a decreased CO at the same end-diastolic volume). Causes of negative inotropic effects include:

➤ hypoxia
➤ myocardial disease (e.g. cardiomyopathies, ischaemic events)
➤ drugs (e.g. flecainide, calcium channel blockers, β-blockers).

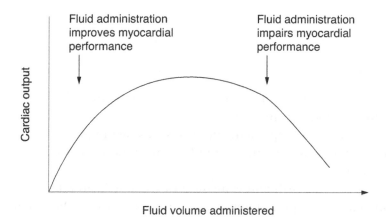

FIGURE 2.10 Effect of fluid resuscitation on cardiac output based on Starling's Law

Cardiac conduction

The anatomy of the cardiac conduction system has been discussed in detail in the section Basic Cardiac Anatomy (*see* page 10).

It is important to understand a few key physiological concepts, as follows.

➤ The sinoatrial node has an inherent spontaneous rate of depolarisation, which varies with age (getting slower with increasing age). It is the SAN that determines the heart rate, with some extrinsic factors also playing a role.
➤ The second pacemaker, the atrioventricular node, acts as a time delay to allow the atria to depolarise and contract first, before the ventricles. This time delay is represented by the PR interval on the ECG.
➤ The AVN also has an inherent spontaneous rate of depolarisation, but this is much slower than the SAN. Therefore, if the SAN is dysfunctional the AVN will take over in control of the heart rate, albeit at a slower rate and with a different morphology of QRS on the ECG depending on the clinical situation.

Control of heart rate

In children, heart rate varies with age, metabolic demand, physical activity and surface area. Table 2.1 lists the normal heart rates for children, but remember that these will change with pain, anxiety, temperature and activity level.

TABLE 2.1 Paediatric heart rate reference ranges

Age of child (years)	Heart rate range (beats per minute)
Under 1	110–160
1–2	100–150
2–5	95–140
5–12	80–120
Over 12	60–100

Physiological factors that determine heart rate include the following.
➤ Vagal nerve activity (cranial nerve X):
  ➤ increase in parasympathetic supply – slows heart rate
  ➤ decrease in parasympathetic supply – increases heart rate.
➤ Medications:
  ➤ β-blockers, anti-arrhythmic medications – slow heart rate
  ➤ salbutamol, atropine, adrenaline, inotropes – increase heart rate.
➤ Hormonal influences:
  ➤ adrenaline and other catecholamines, thyroxine – increase heart rate.
➤ Environmental factors:
  ➤ hypothermia, sleep, increasing age – slow heart rate
  ➤ high temperatures, physical activity, stress, younger age – increases heart rate.

Control of blood pressure

Blood pressure (BP) is a measurement that is not performed in children as much as in adults. However, it still provides much useful information and should be taken seriously.

BP can be calculated using the following formula:

$$BP = [Stroke\ Volume \times Heart\ Rate] \times Peripheral\ Vascular\ Resistance$$

It can be seen that BP is related to cardiac output (SV × HR) and the body's peripheral vascular resistance. Many of the factors that control BP are therefore similar to all the concepts discussed in this chapter so far. Unfortunately, BP control is more complex than this, and its control is heavily influenced by other organs outside the cardiovascular system (including renal, endocrine and neurological systems).

Figure 2.11 displays the interaction in BP control, demonstrating how homeostasis of BP is maintained.

Ranges of BP are variable in children; references exist with centile charts for use (*see* Appendix).

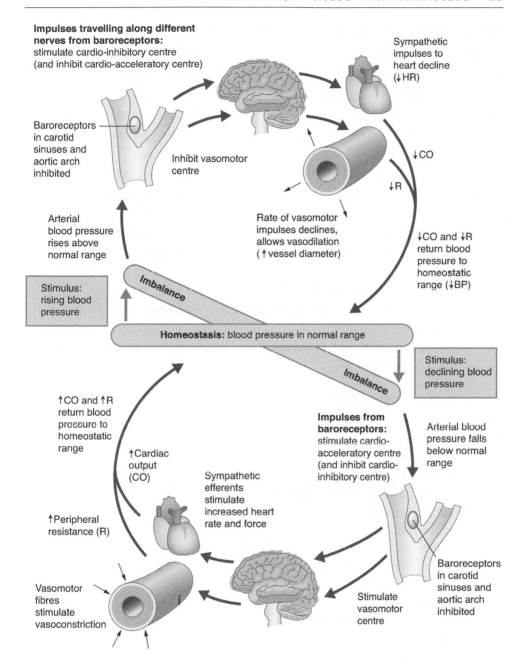

Impulses travelling along different nerves from baroreceptors:
stimulate cardio-inhibitory centre (and inhibit cardio-acceleratory centre)

Sympathetic impulses to heart decline (↓HR)

Baroreceptors in carotid sinuses and aortic arch inhibited

Inhibit vasomotor centre

↓CO

↓R

Arterial blood pressure rises above normal range

Rate of vasomotor impulses declines, allows vasodilation (↑vessel diameter)

↓CO and ↓R return blood pressure to homeostatic range (↓BP)

Stimulus: rising blood pressure

Imbalance

Homeostasis: blood pressure in normal range

Imbalance

Stimulus: declining blood pressure

↑CO and ↑R return blood pressure to homeostatic range

↑Cardiac output (CO)

Sympathetic efferents stimulate increased heart rate and force

Impulses from baroreceptors:
stimulate cardio-acceleratory centre (and inhibit cardio-inhibitory centre)

Arterial blood pressure falls below normal range

↑Peripheral resistance (R)

Vasomotor fibres stimulate vasoconstriction

Stimulate vasomotor centre

Baroreceptors in carotid sinuses and aortic arch inhibited

FIGURE 2.11 Multi-organ control of blood pressure

Common receptor sites and their actions

There are many receptor sites in the heart and blood vessels that provide targets for our medical treatments. Table 2.2 below shows the receptors, common locations and the effect when activated/stimulated (i.e. inhibition will have the opposite effect).

TABLE 2.2 Receptors, sites and actions when stimulated

Receptor	Location	Action when stimulated
α1	Arterioles	Vasoconstriction
α2	Arterioles and coronary circulation	Vasoconstriction
β1	Sinoatrial node	Increase heart rate
	Ventricular muscle	Increase contractility
	Arterioles	Vasodilatation
β2	Sinoatrial node	Increase heart rate
	Ventricular muscle	Increase contractility
	Arterioles	Vasodilatation
	Bronchial smooth muscle	Smooth muscle relaxation
D1 & D2	Peripheral blood vessels	Vasodilatation

BASIC CARDIAC PHARMACOLOGY

A wide range of medications are used in paediatric cardiology and should always be used under expert guidance. For up-to-date indications, contraindications, interactions and drug doses refer to the *British National Formulary* for children or the neonatal formulary.

Classification of drugs groups

Positive inotropic drugs
➤ β-agonists
  ➢ dobutamine
  ➢ adrenaline (epinephrine)
  ➢ noradrenaline (norepinephrine)
➤ D-receptor agonists
  ➢ dopamine
➤ α-agonists
  ➢ noradrenaline (norepinephrine)
➤ cardiac glycosides
  ➢ digoxin
➤ phosphodiesterase inhibitors
  ➢ milrinone
  ➢ enoximone

Diuretics
➤ loop diuretics
  ➢ furosemide
  ➢ bumetanide
➤ thiazides
  ➢ bendroflumethiazide

➤ osmotic
  ➤ mannitol
➤ potassium sparing and aldosterone antagonists
  ➤ spironolactone
➤ carbonic anhydrase inhibitors
  ➤ acetazolamide

Anti-arrhythmic drugs

Anti-arrhythmic drugs can be classified according to their effects on the electrical behaviour of myocardial cells (often these drugs have more than one action).

Vaughan Williams classification:
➤ **Class 1 (sodium channel blockers):** lidocaine, flecainide.
➤ **Class 2 (β-blockers):** atenolol, propranolol.
➤ **Class 3 (potassium channel blockers):** amiodarone, sotalol.
➤ **Class 4 (calcium channel blockers):** verapamil, nifedipine.

Angiotensin converting inhibitors
➤ Captopril
➤ Lisinopril
➤ Enalapril

Angiotensin 2 receptor antagonists
➤ Losartan

β-blockers
➤ Atenolol
➤ Propranolol
➤ Sotalol
➤ Metoprolol

Calcium channel blockers
➤ Nifedipine
➤ Verapamil
➤ Diltiazem

A to Z of common drugs

Drug	**Adenosine**
Class	Anti-arrhythmic drug
Indication	Used to terminate supraventricular tachycardias including Wolff–Parkinson–White syndrome. Also used to aid diagnosis of supraventricular arrhythmias.
Mechanism of action	Acts on the SA and AV nodes and slows conduction through the AV node, lowering heart rate. Adenosine produces many effects which are mediated by two receptors, A1 and A2, which act to increase or decrease intracellular cyclic adenosine monophosphate (cAMP).
Side-effects	Nausea, arrhythmia, angina, dizziness, headache, dyspnoea, flushing.
Contraindications	Second or third-degree heart block, sick sinus syndrome, long QT syndrome, asthma, atrial fibrillation with Wolff–Parkinson–White.
Interactions	Competitively antagonised by methylxanthines (caffeine, theophylline) as they block adenosine receptors. Adenosine uptake is blocked by dipyridamole.
Notes	Should be administered via rapid venous injection into a large central or peripheral vein. Adenosine has a very short duration of action, and side-effects are usually transient.

Drug	**Adrenaline (epinephrine)**
Class	Vasoconstrictor sympathomimetic
Indication	Acute hypotension, CPR – cardiac arrest, anaphylaxis, open angle glaucoma.
Mechanism of action	Acts on alpha and beta receptors, used mainly for its inotropic action. It is produced in some neurons of the central nervous system (CNS) and in the chromaffin cells of the adrenal medulla. In low dose it causes systemic and pulmonary vasodilation, with increase in heart rate, stroke volume and improved contractility (beta receptor). In high dose it causes intense systemic vasoconstriction (mainly alpha receptors).
Side-effects	Nausea and vomiting, dry mouth, palpitations, tachycardia, cold extremities, pulmonary oedema (in overdose).
Contraindications	Closed angle glaucoma.
Interactions	Alcohol, general anaesthetic, β-blockers, antidepressants.
Notes	Can be given via an endotracheal tube (ETT) if no IV access during CPR.

Drug	**Amiodarone hydrochloride**
Class	Anti-arrhythmic agent – class III
Indication	Ventricular tachyarrhythmias, supraventricular arrhythmias. Also used in cardiopulmonary resuscitation (CPR) for ventricular fibrillation (VF) or pulseless ventricular tachycardia (VT) unresponsive to DC shock.
Mechanism of action	Amiodarone prolongs phase 3 of the cardiac action potential, the repolarisation phase. It also acts on the SA and AV nodes, increasing the refractory period via sodium and potassium channel effects and slows intracardiac conduction.

Drug	Amiodarone hydrochloride
Side-effects	Corneal microdeposits – reversible, thyroid dysfunction – hypothyroidism, pneumonitis, nausea and vomiting, taste disturbances, peripheral neuropathy, photosensitivity.
Contraindications	Sinus bradycardia, thyroid dysfunction, iodine sensitivity, pregnancy and breast feeding.
Interactions	β-blockers, digoxin; amiodarone inhibits the metabolism of phenytoin and warfarin.
Notes	Amiodarone has a very long half-life. Many weeks to months may be required to achieve steady-state plasma amiodarone concentration. It is fat soluble. Available in oral and intravenous (IV) preparations.

Drug	Atenolol
Class	Beta 1 blocker
Indication	Hypertension, angina, SVT/VT, long QT syndrome, secondary prophylaxis of myocardial infarction (MI), thyrotoxicosis, migraine prophylaxis.
Mechanism of action	Atenolol is a selective beta 1 receptor antagonist. It blocks the beta-adrenoceptors in the heart, peripheral vasculature, bronchi, pancreas and liver. It is water soluble and excreted by the kidneys. Atenolol has a half-life of around 6 hours; it hydrophilic. It is cardioselective but not cardio-specific.
Side-effects	Bradycardia, gastrointestinal (GI) disturbances, hypotension, hypoglycaemia, peripheral vasoconstriction, fatigue, cold extremities, sleep disturbances.
Contraindications	Bradycardia, cardiogenic shock, asthma, sick sinus syndrome, phaeochromocytoma.
Interactions	Verapamil – risk of hypotension and asystole.
Notes	β-blockers can affect carbohydrate metabolism causing both hypo- and hyperglycaemia. They may mask the symptoms of hypoglycaemia and should be avoided in children with recurrent hypoglycaemia episodes.

Drug	Atropine
Class	Antimuscarinic drug
Indication	CPR, bradycardia, premedication, cycloplegia.
Mechanism of action	Atropine increases conduction through the SA and AV node of the heart, increasing heart rate. It blocks acetylcholine receptor sites and decreases bronchial secretions. It decreases activity of the parasympathetic nervous system. It is a competitive antagonist of the muscarinic acetylcholine receptors. Atropine blocks the action of the vagus nerve. It is a part of the parasympathetic system whose main action is to decrease heart rate.
Side-effects	Dry mouth, confusion, blurred vision, hallucinations, constipation.
Contraindications	Prostatic hypertrophy, closed angle glaucoma.
Interactions	Antidepressants may potentiate anticholinergic side-effects of atropine.
Notes	Atropine crosses the blood–brain barrier (BBB). It has a half-life of 2 hours.

Drug	Bosentan
Class	Vasodilator
Indication	Idiopathic pulmonary arterial hypertension.
Mechanism of action	A dual endothelin receptor antagonist. It is a competitive antagonist of endothelin-1 at the endothelin A and B receptors.
	Bosentan decreases pulmonary vascular resistance.
Side-effects	GI disturbances, dry mouth, flushing, hypotension.
Contraindications	Acute porphyria, hepatic impairment, pregnancy – teratogenic, breast feeding.
Interactions	Rifampicin, fluconazole, simvastatin, sildenafil.
Notes	Monitor liver function test (LFT) and haemoglobin (Hb) before treatment and at monthly intervals.

Drug	Captopril
Class	Angiotensin-converting enzyme inhibitor
Indication	Heart failure, hypertension, diabetic nephropathy, post MI.
Mechanism of action	Captopril decreases the conversion of angiotensin I to angiotensin II. Decreased levels of angiotensin II lead to decreased peripheral resistance, decreased peripheral vasoconstriction and less sodium and water retention. This in turn improves ventricular emptying and improves cardiac function.
Side-effects	Profound hypotension, renal impairment, rash, persistent dry cough, angioedema.
Contraindications	Bilateral renovascular disease, pregnancy.
Interactions	Diuretics, non-steroidal anti-inflammatory drugs (NSAIDs) – increased risk of renal impairment.
Notes	About 70% of oral captopril is absorbed.

Drug	Chlorothiazide
Class	Thiazide diuretic
Indication	Heart failure, hypertension, ascites.
Mechanism of action	Chlorothiazide inhibits sodium reabsorption at the start of the distal collecting tubule.
Side-effects	GI disturbances, postural hypotension, hypokalaemia, hyponatraemia.
Contraindications	Renal failure, hypokalaemia/hyponatraemia, Addison's disease.
Interactions	None.
Notes	Should be used with caution in hepatic and renal impairment.

Drug	Digoxin
Class	Cardiac glycoside
Indication	Atrial fibrillation, atrial flutter, chronic heart failure, supraventricular tachycardias.
Mechanism of action	It is a purified cardiac glycoside extracted from the foxglove plant, *Digitalis lanata*. It increases the force of myocardial contraction and reduced conductivity within the AV node.
Side-effects	Nausea and vomiting, diarrhoea, dizziness, blurred or yellow vision.
Contraindications	Complete heart block, second-degree heart block, WPW (can be used in infancy), VT/VF.
Interactions	Calcium channel blockers, diuretics.
Notes	Intramuscular (IM) route is not recommended. Hypokalaemia predisposes the child to digitalis toxicity. Digoxin has a narrow therapeutic index and plasma-digoxin concentration should be monitored.

Drug	Dobutamine
Class	Inotropic sympathomimetic
Indication	Heart failure, cardiogenic shock, septic shock.
Mechanism of action	Dobutamine is a cardiac stimulant acting on beta receptors in cardiac muscle, increasing contractility with little effect on rate. It is predominantly a beta 1 adrenergic agonist with weak beta 2 and alpha 1 selective activity. It is dose dependent.
Side-effects	Hypertension, angina, arrhythmia, tachycardia.
Contraindications	Phaeochromocytoma.
Interactions	None.
Notes	Does not reduce renal perfusion. Often commenced in combination with dopamine.

Drug	Dopamine
Class	Inotropic sympathomimetic
Indication	Severe heart failure, cardiogenic shock.
Mechanism of action	Dopamine has a dose-dependent impact on vascular tone. It is a member of the catecholamine family and is a precursor to noradrenaline and then adrenaline in the biosynthetic pathway.
Side-effects	Nausea and vomiting, peripheral vasoconstriction, hypo/hypertension, tachycardia.
Contraindications	Tachyarrhythmia, phaeochromocytoma.
Interactions	Monoamine oxidase inhibitor.
Notes	Low dose – vasodilation.
	Moderate dose – increased myocardial contractility, increased cardiac output in older children, decreased cardiac output in neonates.
	High doses – vasoconstriction/increased vascular resistance.

Drug	**Flecainide**
Class	Class 1a membrane-stabilising drug
Indication	Resistant re-entry SVT, VT, WPW syndrome, paroxysmal atrial fibrillation (AF), to aid diagnosis of Brugada syndrome.
Mechanism of action	Flecainide regulates the flow of sodium in the heart, causing prolongation of the cardiac action potential. It works by blocking the Nav1.5 sodium channel. This slows conduction within the heart, causing decreased myocardial contractility and decreasing ejection fraction.
Side-effects	Oedema, dyspnoea, fatigue, visual disturbance, pneumonitis, hallucinations.
Contraindications	Heart failure, abnormal LV function, sinus node dysfunction, bundle branch block (BBB).
Interactions	Alcohol, amiodarone, digoxin.
Notes	Crosses the placenta and can be used to treat fetal supraventricular arrhythmias. It has a high oral bioavailability and a narrow therapeutic index.

Drug	**Furosemide**
Class	Loop diuretic
Indication	Congestive heart failure, oedema, hypertension, renal impairment, oliguria.
Mechanism of action	Loop diuretics inhibit reabsorption of sodium, potassium and chloride from the ascending limb of the loop of Henle in the renal tubule. They inhibit the sodium/potassium/chloride pump. This leads to increase in salt, water and potassium excretion reducing cardiac preload.
Side-effects	Mild GI disturbances, pancreatitis, postural hypotension, hyperglycaemia.
Contraindications	Hepatic/renal impairment; may precipitate hepatic encephalopathy.
Interactions	Antibacterials, digoxin, lithium.
Notes	Loop diuretics can exacerbate diabetes and gout.

Drug	**Lidocaine hydrochloride**
Class	Class 1b membrane-stabilising drug
Indication	CPR – VF or pulseless VT unresponsive to DC shock, congestive heart failure, acute MI, digitalis poisoning.
Mechanism of action	It is metabolised in the liver by CYP3A4 to active metabolite monoethylglycinexylidide (MEGX) which is a sodium channel blocker.
Side-effects	Dizziness, paraesthesia, drowsiness, confusion, respiratory depression.
Contraindications	Sinoatrial disorders, AV block, severe myocardial depression, acute porphyria.
Interactions	Antibacterials, β-blockers, muscle relaxants.
Notes	Crosses the placenta but not thought to be harmful.

Drug	**Milrinone**
Class	Phosphodiesterase inhibitors
Indication	Congestive heart failure, low cardiac output especially after cardiac surgery, shock.
Mechanism of action	Milrinone is a selective phosphodiesterase 3 inhibitor. It potentiates the effect of cAMP. It has positive inotropic and vasodilator properties.
Side-effects	Ectopic beats, hypotension, headache, nausea and vomiting, ventricular arrhythmias.
Contraindications	Renal impairment, pregnancy, breast feeding.
Interactions	Anagrelide (a treatment from thrombocytosis).
Notes	Long-term oral administration has been associated with increased mortality in adults in congestive heart failure.

Drug	**Noradrenaline**
Class	Vasoconstrictor sympathomimetic
Indication	Acute hypotension, septic shock, spinal shock, anaphylaxis.
Mechanism of action	The actions of noradrenaline are mediated via the binding to adrenergic receptors. It is synthesised from dopamine by dopamine beta hydroxylase and released from the adrenal medulla. It acts on alpha 1 and alpha 2 adrenergic receptors to cause vasoconstriction, increasing systemic vascular resistance.
Side-effects	Hypertension, bradycardia, headache, peripheral ischaemia.
Contraindications	Hypertension, pregnancy – may reduce placental perfusion.
Interactions	Alcohol, general anaesthesia, β-blockers.
Notes	Used in children with low systemic vascular resistance unresponsive to fluid resuscitation.

Drug	**Nitric oxide**
Class	Pulmonary vasodilator
Indication	Pulmonary arterial hypertension, *persistent pulmonary hypertension of the newborn*.
Mechanism of action	Nitric oxide is a binary molecule known as the endothelium-derived relaxing factor. It signals to smooth muscle, causing smooth muscle relaxation, vasodilation and increased blood flow. Nitric oxide acts on cyclic guanosine monophosphate (cGMP), resulting in smooth muscle relaxation.
Side-effects	Methaemoglobinaemia as a result of excess nitric oxide. Increased risk of haemorrhage.
Contraindications	None.
Interactions	None.
Notes	Rebound pulmonary hypertension may occur if nitric oxide is stopped abruptly. Sildenafil may be used to gradually withdraw nitric oxide.

Drug	Prostaglandins
Class	Vasodilators
	Prostaglandin E1 – alprostadil
	Prostaglandin E2 – dinoprostone
Indication	Maintain the patency of the ductus arteriosus.
Mechanism of action	PGE2 is generated from the action of prostaglandin E synthesis on prostaglandin H2. Prostaglandins are found in most tissues and organs, produced by nucleated cells they are synthesised from essential fatty acids.
Side-effects	Apnoea, pyrexia, profound bradycardia, hypotension, flushing, cardiac arrest, prolonged use – gastric outlet obstruction.
Contraindications	None.
Interactions	ACE inhibitors, alpha blockers, β-blockers, calcium channel blockers.
Notes	Recurrent or prolonged apnoeas may require ventilatory support.
	The side effects are dose related.

Drug	Sildenafil
Class	Selective phosphodiesterase type 5 inhibitor
Indication	Pulmonary arterial hypertension, erectile dysfunction.
Mechanism of action	It acts by inhibiting cGMP-specific phosphodiesterase type 5. It relaxes the arterial wall, leading to decreased pulmonary arterial resistance and pressure, which in turn reduces the workload of the RV. It is metabolised by liver enzymes and excreted by both the liver and the kidneys.
Side-effects	Headache, flushing, blurred vision, severe hypotension, MI, priapism.
Contraindications	Severe hepatic and renal impairment, nitrites and nitrates – glyceryl trinitrate (GTN).
Interactions	Protease inhibitors, β-blockers.
Notes	Sildenafil has been used to wean children off inhaled nitric oxide following cardiac surgery.

Drug	Spironolactone
Class	Aldosterone antagonist
Indication	Heart failure, ascites, hypertension, nephritic syndrome, Bartter syndrome, polycystic ovarian syndrome (PCOS).
Mechanism of action	Spironolactone is the most commonly used potassium-sparing diuretic in children. On its own spironolactone is a weak diuretic because it primarily targets the distal collecting tubule. It enhances potassium retention and sodium excretion in the distal collecting tubule. It has an anti-androgen effect and can be used to treat PCOS.
Side-effects	Gynaecomastia in males, GI disturbances, hepatotoxicity, menstrual disturbances, hyperkalaemia.

Drug	Spironolactone
Contraindications	Hyperkalaemia, hyponatraemia, Addison's disease.
Interactions	Antidepressants.
Notes	Spironolactone has a slow onset of action.

Drug	Verapamil hydrochloride
Class	Calcium channel blocker, Class IV anti-arrhythmic agent
Indication	Hypertension, atrial tachyarrhythmias, angina pectoris.
Mechanism of action	Verapamil is a highly negatively inotropic calcium channel blocker. It blocks voltage-dependent calcium channels. It decreases impulse conduction through the AV node, reduces cardiac output and slows the heart rate. Verapamil inhibits the influx of calcium into smooth muscle, resulting in smooth muscle relaxation. It has a half-life of 5–12 hours and is metabolised in the liver to inactive metabolites.
Side-effects	Hypotension, constipation, nausea and vomiting, flushing, headache, ankle swelling.
Contraindications	Hypotension, bradycardia, pregnancy, second/third-degree AV block, sick sinus syndrome, acute porphyria, VT.
Interactions	β-blockers – increase risk of severe hypotension, asystole and heart failure. Digoxin.
Notes	It may precipitate heart failure.

CHAPTER 3

Examination of the cardiovascular system

Inspection
Palpation
Percussion
Auscultation

The cardiovascular system should be examined using the same principle as for examining other systems:
➤ inspection
➤ palpation
➤ percussion
➤ auscultation.

Examining any child requires practice, patience and skill. It is essential to gain the child's confidence; distraction often works very well. Although we are traditionally taught to examine using a systematic approach, with very young children this is not always possible and you need to tailor the examination to the needs of the child.

INSPECTION

General

Look at the child as a whole. Does the child look well or unwell? Undress the child as appropriate to the age and pubertal stage of development. Involving the parents/carers of very young children can be very helpful. Inspect for:
➤ general health
➤ nutritional status
➤ dysmorphic features
➤ colour: cyanosis, pallor
➤ surgical scars.

Face

Look specifically at the child's face: is the child cyanotic, indicating more than 5 g/dL of desaturated blood in the capillaries? It can be difficult to detect by the naked eye. Offer to measure the oxygen saturation using a pulse oximeter. The child may be polycythaemic, a state seen in children with congenital heart disease and a raised haematocrit level.

Mouth

Look at the level of oral hygiene, and if appropriate comment on the importance of dental care in association with certain cardiac conditions. Comment on the colour of the oral mucosae.

Hands

Always look for healed cannulation scars along with:
➤ clubbing
➤ splinter haemorrhages
➤ Osler's nodes
➤ bony abnormalities which may indicate a specific syndrome.

Praecordium

Get the child to lift both arms up and inspect the entire praecordium for surgical scars, including scars from a chest drain:
➤ right thoracotomy scar
➤ left thoracotomy scar
➤ midline sternotomy
➤ chest drains
➤ IV access – Hickman lines
➤ additional abdominal/renal scars.

Count the respiratory rate and comment on any apparent chest wall deformities.

PALPATION
Pulses

Palpate peripheral and central pulses:
➤ radial
➤ brachial
➤ femoral.

Are the pulses present or absent? An absent radial pulse may be a congenital malformation, or postoperative (e.g. repair of coarctation with subclavian flap), whereas an absent femoral pulse is associated with coarctation of the aorta. Radiofemoral delay can be difficult to detect clinically in a child but should be commented upon.

Comment on:

➤ rate
➤ rhythm
➤ volume
➤ character.

TABLE 3.1 Normal resting heart rates in children

Age of child	Beats per minute
Less than 12 months	110–160
2–5 years	95–140
5–12 years	80–120
Over 12 years	60–100

Palpate the **apex beat**: fourth to fifth intercostal space in the mid-clavicular line. Always comment on the position of the apex beat: a displacement to the left may indicate underlying cardiomegaly, while an apex beat displaced to the right side may be due to dextrocardia.

Thrill

A palpable murmur equates to grade 4–6 murmur. Palpate the suprasternal notch gently to detect the thrill found in aortic stenosis.

Heave

A parasternal heave felt at the lower left sternal edge would indicate a right ventricular hypertrophy.

Jugular venous pressure

This does not form a routine part of the cardiovascular examination in children, but it would be raised in right-sided heart failure and pericardial tamponade.

PERCUSSION

You can palpate the outline of the cardiac border. However, this is rarely helpful in children.

AUSCULTATION

After auscultating the four main areas: (1) aortic area; (2) pulmonary area; (3) tricuspid area; (4) mitral/apex area (*see* Figure 3.1); comment upon:

➤ heart sounds
➤ added sounds
➤ murmurs.

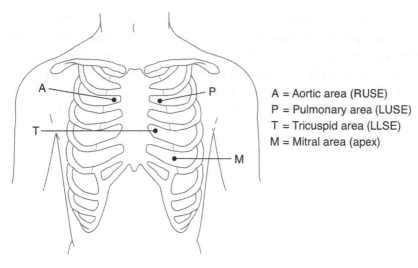

A = Aortic area (RUSE)
P = Pulmonary area (LUSE)
T = Tricuspid area (LLSE)
M = Mitral area (apex)

FIGURE 3.1 Auscultation areas

First heart sound
Closure of first the mitral valve, followed by the tricuspid valve.

Second heart sound
Closure of the aortic valve, followed by closure of the pulmonary valve.

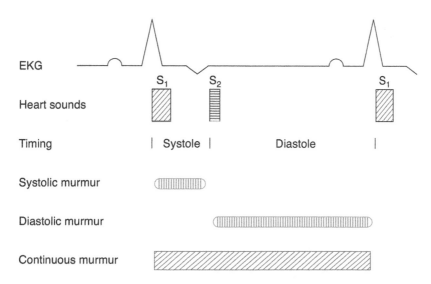

FIGURE 3.2 Grading and timing of cardiac murmurs: a schematic diagram

Systolic murmurs are graded from 1 to 6, with grade 4 if a thrill is palpable. Diastolic murmurs are graded from 1 to 4.

For specific details of murmurs *see* pages 139–42.

Always conclude your examination by offering to plot the child's height and weight on an appropriate growth chart, and to measure the blood pressure. To complete any cardiovascular examination you should routinely palpate the abdomen, feeling specifically for organomegaly. Hepatomegaly is an important sign of heart failure, particularly in infants. If appropriate you may go on to perform urinalysis, fundoscopy and determine the child's developmental level.

CHAPTER 4

Interpretation of the paediatric ECG

Introduction
What does each wave and segment represent?
Check the demographic data of the child
Check technical settings on ECG
Are the machine-generated values correct?
Calculate the heart rate
Assess the rhythm
Assess for regularity
Calculate the frontal (QRS) axis
Assess the P waves
Assess the QRS complex
Assess the T waves
Assess the ST segments
Assess the PR interval
Assess the QT interval
Formulate a conclusion
Paediatric ECG reference ranges

INTRODUCTION

ECG interpretation in children is not as scary as it seems! The key to successful interpretation is to follow a logical structure, documenting each finding as you go. The sequence of interpretation of the ECG is demonstrated in Figure 4.1.

WHAT DOES EACH WAVE AND SEGMENT REPRESENT?

Understanding what each part of the ECG signifies will help with your interpretation of the ECG you are facing. Figure 4.2 displays the names of the waves, intervals and segments that are often seen in children and adults.

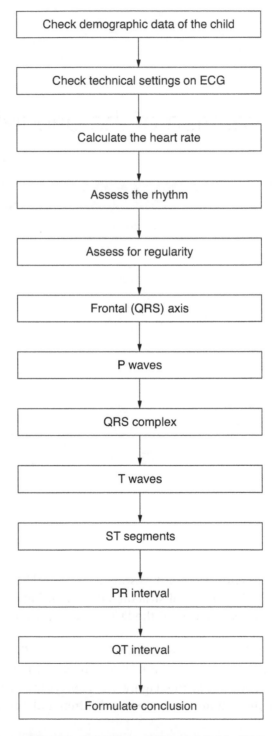

FIGURE 4.1 Sequence for interpretation of the paediatric ECG

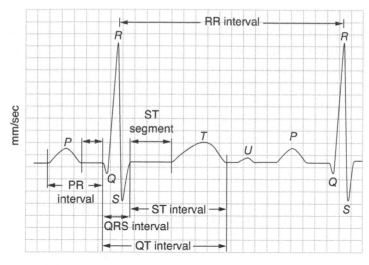

mm/mV   1 square = 0.04 sec/0.1mV

FIGURE 4.2 ECG wave, interval and segment identification

Waves
➤ P wave = atrial depolarisation.
➤ QRS complex = ventricular depolarisation (also masking atrial repolarisation).
➤ T wave = ventricular repolarisation.
➤ U wave = insignificant finding on the ECG of little consequence and not always present. Thought to represent repolarisation of the Purkinje fibres or papillary muscles, although this has not been proven.

Intervals
➤ PR interval = time for transmission of impulse through the AV node.
➤ QT interval = time taken for ventricular depolarisation and repolarisation to occur.
➤ ST interval = time for ventricular repolarisation to occur.
➤ RR interval = time between one ventricular beat and the next.

CHECK THE DEMOGRAPHIC DATA OF THE CHILD
The first question to ask when reviewing a paediatric ECG is how old the child is, as the normal values for many variables are age dependent. This is discussed in more detail in each section below. A table of normal values for age can be found in the Appendix.

CHECK TECHNICAL SETTINGS ON ECG

As with adult ECGs, check that the ECG paper speed is set at 25 mm/s and the sensitivity is 10 mm/mV for both limb and chest leads. There should be a calibration square which is 10 mm high (i.e. 1 mV) and 5 mm wide at the start or end of the rhythm strip. With these settings you can calculate that a 1 mm block or box (i.e. one small square) is 0.04 seconds in duration, and a 5 mm block (i.e. one large square) is 0.2 seconds in duration. This is demonstrated in Figure 4.3.

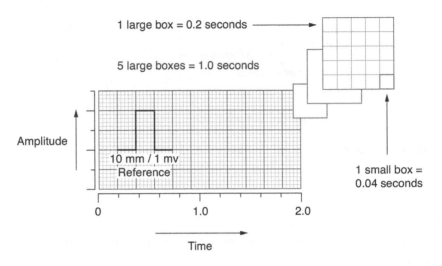

FIGURE 4.3 Technical settings on the ECG

This is particularly important in children; ECGs are sometimes documented on 'half scale'. Usually, the person recording the ECG should document this on the ECG itself. However, it can be recognised by the fact the calibration square is only 5 mm high (i.e. 0.5 mV).

A filter frequency value will often be printed on the ECG (around 50 Hz), which is important as it filters out electrical interference (e.g. from lights).

ARE THE MACHINE-GENERATED VALUES CORRECT?

Many ECG machines will calculate the following parameters we are about to discuss, and usually will print them on the top left corner of the ECG. Furthermore, some ECGs will also give you an analysis.

Be cautious with paediatric ECGs; many of the standard ECGs analyse the ECG against adult pre-sets and so the written report is often incorrect. Some machines have a paediatric ECG analytical program. The values printed are usually accurate, and should be taken seriously if deranged, but you should always confirm these values by manual calculations.

CALCULATE THE HEART RATE

Heart rate is age dependent. Many different methods exist for calculating heart rate from the ECG. Each has advantages and disadvantages. The following are three commonly used methods.

1 300/number of large squares between one R-R interval.
2 1500/number of small squares between one R-R interval.
3 Assuming a calibration square is present on a standard 12-lead ECG rhythm strip, you will know that the rhythm strip is recorded over 10 seconds. Therefore each QRS complex represents one beat and so heart rate (beats per minute) can be calculated by multiplying the number of QRS complexes in this rhythm strip by 6.

The definitions of tachycardia (rapid heart rate) and bradycardia (slow heart rate) will vary depending on the age of the child.

ASSESS THE RHYTHM

A rhythm can be classified as a sinus rhythm or non-sinus rhythm.

For an ECG to be described as sinus rhythm in a child the following criteria must be met.

➤ A P wave precedes every QRS complex.
➤ This P wave must be upright in limb leads I and II (i.e. a normal P-wave axis).
➤ The heart rate must be within an age-appropriate range.

ASSESS FOR REGULARITY

Regularity of the QRS complexes can be checked by marking three QRS complexes on a separate piece of paper, and moving these markers along the rhythm strip, ensuring a QRS complex is present at each predicted location of the markers.

Children often display sinus arrhythmia. This is the phenomenon where the heart rate increases on inspiration and decreases on expiration. As a result, the R-R interval is variable and so the ECG can appear to be irregular. This is normal. Sinus arrhythmia is lost when the child is upset/nervous/unwell.

Unlike in adults, truly irregular QRS complexes in children are rare. If present in a child, an irregular QRS complex usually suggests atrial flutter with a variable AV conduction block or a form of atrial tachycardia or atrial fibrillation.

CALCULATE THE FRONTAL (QRS) AXIS

The term frontal axis is used to describe the overall direction (net vector) of the electrical impulses within the heart. It provides a great deal of information and is important in paediatric ECG interpretation.

It is important to understand that the axis changes with age. A neonate has a very dominant right ventricle, and so a greater proportion of the electrically conducted impulses will go to the right side. As the child gets older the left ventricle becomes more dominant, and so the axis will slowly change with age. Once again, reference ranges are important. This concept is demonstrated in Figure 4.4.

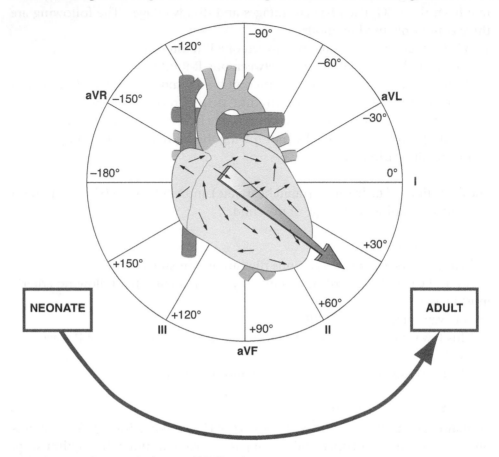

FIGURE 4.4 Change in frontal (QRS) axis

Having understood the definition of frontal cardiac axis, it is now important to calculate it. This is not as difficult as people first think! Many different methods exist for calculating the axis. All come with a similar answer. However, one of the methods is discussed below and requires a 'working out' approach, rather than a detailed understanding of the isoelectric lead method.

1 Identify lead I and aVF on the 12-lead ECG. These leads are selected as they view the heart at a 90-degree angle to one another (*see* Figure 4.4).

2 On the ECG find an area with spare grid paper, and draw grid lines as demonstrated in Figure 4.5A. Sometimes the ECG will print this graph out for you.

3 The x-axis will represent lead I and the y-axis will represent aVF. By convention, lead I looks at the heart at 0 degrees. Lead aVF looks at the heart at 90 degrees. This is shown in Figure 4.5B. (Remember, electrical impulses moving towards the lead give a positive deflection; impulses moving away give a negative deflection.)

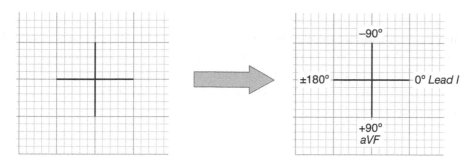

FIGURE 4.5A, B Preparing to calculate frontal QRS axis

4 You then need to calculate the net vector of lead I. This is calculated by subtracting the negative deflection (Q+S) from the positive deflection (R wave). This is demonstrated in Figure 4.5C. Do the same for aVF (Figure 4.5D).

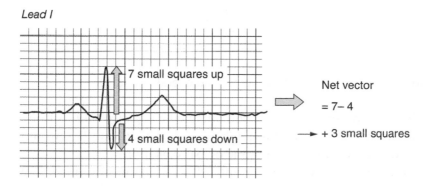

FIGURE 4.5C Calculating the net vector of lead I

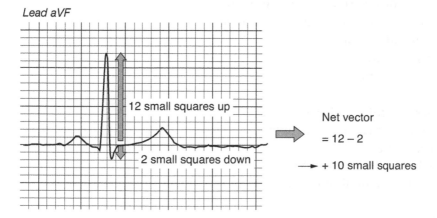

FIGURE 4.5D Calculating the net vector of lead aVF

5 You can now plot your values on the graph you made earlier. So for lead I, you mark 3 small squares along the x-axis, towards lead I (as it is a positive value). For lead aVF you plot 10 small squares along the y-axis downwards towards aVF (as it is a positive value). You join the dots, and the angle formed by the vector is your frontal QRS axis. This is shown in Figure 4.5E. In this case, the net axis is around 55 to 60 degrees.

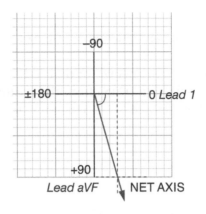

FIGURE 4.5E Calculating the net vector and overall frontal axis

Note that if in the above example you obtained a negative value for one of your calculations, you would plot the graph away from that lead. This would change the net axis and would be an example of axis deviation.

We describe axis deviation as right, left or extreme/superior (greater than 180 degrees). The axis deviation for age can give you an indicator as to the underlying diagnosis.

Causes of superior axis deviation are:
➤ complete atrioventricular septal defect
➤ tricuspid atresia
➤ Ebstein's anomaly
➤ Noonan syndrome.

Causes of right axis deviation are:
➤ right ventricular hypertrophy
➤ dextrocardia
➤ right bundle branch block
➤ secundum atrial septal defect.

Causes of left axis deviation are:
➤ left ventricular hypertrophy
➤ left bundle branch block
➤ partial AVSD.

ASSESS THE P WAVES

P waves represent atrial depolarisation. They are best visualised in leads II and VI. The P waves give useful information about both atrial structure and function.

The normal P wave should be upright in leads I and II and no more than 2.5 mm high in children (up to 3 mm is acceptable in under 6 months) and no wider than 2 to 2.5 mm. The P wave can be biphasic in lead V1. The P waves should all look the same throughout the rhythm strip within the same lead. Variable P-wave morphology can suggest a multifocal atrial tachycardia, and further advice should be sought.

An inverted P wave in lead I or II suggests one of the following:
➤ limb leads incorrectly positioned
➤ dextrocardia
➤ non-sinus node generated rhythm (e.g. a form of atrioventricular re-entry tachycardia known as permanent junctional reciprocating tachycardia)
➤ post-cardiac surgery
➤ left atrial isomerism (i.e. two left atria and no right atria, hence no SA node so atrial depolarisation has to occur at a different site to normal).

A peaked P wave over 3 mm high (also known as P-pulmonale, *see* Figure 4.6) suggests right atrial hypertrophy, which can be caused by many things, including:
➤ pulmonary hypertension
➤ Ebstein's anomaly
➤ severe tricuspid regurgitation
➤ cardiomyopathy.

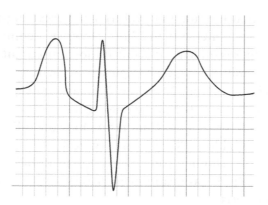

FIGURE 4.6 P-pulmonale, suggesting right atrial hypertrophy

A wide, often bifid P wave longer than 2 mm wide (also known as P-mitrale; *see* Figure 4.7) suggests left atrial hypertrophy, which can be caused by:
➤ mitral stenosis
➤ severe mitral regurgitation
➤ cardiomyopathy.

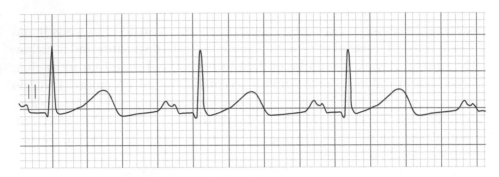

FIGURE 4.7 P-mitrale, suggesting left atrial hypertrophy

It is very rare that P waves are absent from an ECG trace, even in SVT. More often, the P wave is hidden within the QRS complex. SVT is a non-specific term, and will be discussed later; however, the P waves can give useful information into the type of SVT. This is out of the scope of this book, and readers are recommended to consult a textbook on paediatric arrhythmias for more details.

ASSESS THE QRS COMPLEX

The QRS complex represents ventricular depolarisation and is often the most prominent wave on the ECG. It represents ventricular contraction (i.e. a ventricular beat). The nomenclature of the QRS complex is simple: the first negative (downward) deflection after the P wave is known as the Q wave, the first positive (upright) deflection is the R wave, and the second negative deflection is the S wave.

It is important to note the duration (width) of the QRS complex. Typically, children have a slightly shorter QRS than adults. However, defining a narrow versus a normal QRS complex is difficult. It is much more important to identify a wide complex QRS. The duration for QRS complexes for each age group can be found at the end of this chapter. Over 120 ms (i.e. 3 small squares) is prolonged in any age group, although this is not always pathological.

The causes of a wide/broad QRS complex include the following.

➤ Right bundle branch block (RBBB) – *see* Figure 4.8A:
  ➢ normal variant in children (often 'incomplete' RBBB)
  ➢ rate-related RBBB (i.e. as heart rate increases RBBB develops)
  ➢ atrial septal defects
  ➢ postoperative (especially with repair of tetralogy of Fallot or large VSD)
  ➢ Brugada syndrome (along with ST elevation in V1/2).
➤ Left bundle branch block (LBBB) – *see* Figure 4.8B:
  ➢ postoperative (especially with aortic valve/left ventricular outlet surgery)
  ➢ rate-related LBBB (i.e. as heart rate increases LBBB develops)
  ➢ aortic stenosis.

➤ Arrhythmia:
  ➤ ventricular tachycardia
  ➤ supraventricular tachycardia with bundle branch block
  ➤ SVT with obvious ventricular pre-excitation (SVT with a delta wave)
  ➤ Wolff–Parkinson–White syndrome in sinus rhythm.
➤ Hyperkalaemia
➤ Certain metabolic disorders (e.g. Pompe disease).

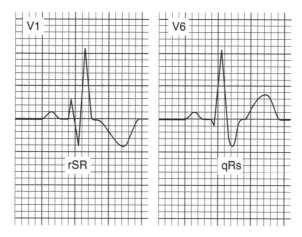

FIGURE 4.8A RBBB seen best in V1 with an RSR pattern and wide QRS

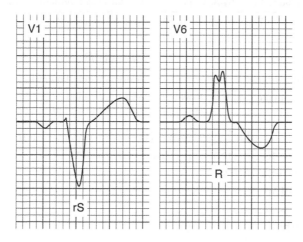

FIGURE 4.8B LBBB seen best in V6 with an RSR pattern and wide QRS

Please note that while we talk about the QRS complex, not all children will have
Q waves. In children, very deep obvious Q waves (when the Q wave is greater in
amplitude than 25% of the associated R wave) can be caused by:
➤ ventricular hypertrophy (left or right)
➤ myocardial infarction (e.g. with ALCAPA defect)

➤ myocardial ischaemia (e.g. with Kawasaki disease)
➤ left ventricular volume overload (e.g. dilated cardiomyopathy, large VSD).

The final point to consider when reviewing the QRS complex is the amplitude. People often use the ECG to look for evidence of ventricular hypertrophy based on QRS amplitude. While the ECG can give an indicator of ventricular hypertrophy, it is important to appreciate that it is *not* the gold standard for hypertrophy assessment; you need an echocardiogram.

Probably the most useful tool for ventricular hypertrophy assessment is to look at the R wave progression throughout leads V1 to V6. V1 looks at the anterior aspect of the heart (the right ventricle) and V6 looks at the lateral aspect of the heart (the left ventricle). V7 and V8 leads can be added to consider the posterior aspect of the heart (the left ventricle again). When the RV is dominant the R wave will be dominant in V1, and get gradually smaller towards V6. In LV dominance the R wave is tallest in V6, and often only small in V1 (with a dominant S wave in V1).

The neonate will have RV dominance (*see* cardiac axis section). Unlike adults, it is difficult to find reliable criteria to diagnose hypertrophy from an ECG in children. The ECG will have some clues for ventricular hypertrophy, as displayed in Table 4.1. Remember – if in doubt, arrange for an echocardiogram.

TABLE 4.1 ECG criteria to suggest ventricular hypertrophy

ECG features suggestive of RV hypertrophy	ECG features suggestive of LV hypertrophy
Upright T wave in V1 (from 7 days to late teenager) – see below	Inverted T wave in V6
Q waves in V1	Q waves in V6
R waves greater than 20 mm in V1	R waves greater than 20 mm in V6
Right axis deviation (with other findings above)	Left axis deviation

Causes of right ventricular hypertrophy (considering age) include:
➤ any obstruction to the right ventricular outflow tract
➤ pulmonary stenosis/atresia
➤ tetralogy of Fallot
➤ pulmonary hypertension
➤ cardiomyopathy.

Causes of left ventricular hypertrophy include:
➤ any obstruction to the left ventricular outflow tract
➤ aortic stenosis
➤ coarctation of the aorta
➤ systemic hypertension (for whatever cause)
➤ cardiomyopathy.

ASSESS THE T WAVES

The T waves follow the QRS, and represent the ventricular repolarisation period. It is important to appreciate that T-wave morphology changes with age. In the first week of life the T wave is upright (positive) in V1–3. It then inverts and becomes a negative wave until adolescence, when it should then become upright.

The significance of this is that a persistently upright T wave is not normal in children, and it is often a sign of right ventricular hypertrophy (*see* Table 4.1).

T waves can provide some useful information about cardiac and non-cardiac conditions based on the T-wave morphology. Table 4.2 demonstrates some situations when T-wave morphology can be helpful.

TABLE 4.2 Types of T-wave morphology and causes

T-wave morphology	Significance
Peaked (high amplitude)	Hyperkalaemia
Flat (low amplitude)	Digoxin related
	Hypokalaemia
	Ischaemia
	Hypothyroidism
Inappropriate T-wave inversion (for age)	Cardiomyopathies
	Digoxin related Myocarditis, Ischaemia, Hypothyroidism
Inappropriate upright T waves (for age)	Right ventricular hypertrophy
Beat-to-beat variation in T-wave morphology (T-wave alternans)	Long QT syndrome

ASSESS THE ST SEGMENTS

The ST segment should be an isoelectric line between the S wave at the end of the QRS to the start of the T wave. Adult physicians are particularly interested in the ST segment as it is often changed in myocardial infarctions. Although rare, similar problems can happen in children.

It is considered normal for the ST segment to be raised 1 mm from the iso-electric baseline in the limb leads and 2 mm from the isoelectric baseline in the chest leads. Any increase over this limit is termed 'ST elevation'. This needs to be carefully distinguished from 'high take-off' due to early repolarisation. In this case, the ST segment is not actually raised; it is simply the T wave that gives this effect at first glance. Examples of ST high take-off are shown in Figure 4.9A and ST elevation in Figure 4.9B.

Causes of ST elevation in paediatric practice include:
➤ pericarditis
➤ Brugada syndrome
➤ acute myocardial infarction (e.g. ALCAPA)
➤ shortly following cardiac surgery.

A

B

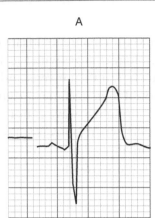
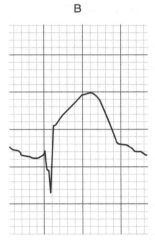

FIGURE 4.9 ST changes: (a) High take-off (b) Genuine elevation

Causes of ST depression in paediatric practice include:
➤ ischaemia (e.g. ALCAPA, Kawasaki disease)
➤ cardiomyopathy
➤ digoxin-related effect
➤ metabolic effects on the heart (e.g. mucopolysaccharidoses, glycogen storage diseases).

ASSESS THE PR INTERVAL
The PR interval represents the time delay between the atrial activity passing through the atrioventricular node to the ventricles. This delay is important to allow atrial contraction before ventricular contraction. It is measured from the start of the P wave to the start of the QRS complex. The PR interval is shorter in a neonate with a progressive increase in time with age.

The PR interval can be prolonged or short. Causes of a prolonged PR interval are:
➤ first-degree heart block (can be normal variant if high vagal tone, such as in athletes)
➤ post-cardiac surgery
➤ atrioventricular septal defects
➤ myocarditis
➤ digoxin toxicity (along with ST depression and inverted/flat T waves)
➤ rheumatic fever
➤ hypokalaemia.

Causes of a short PR interval include:
➤ Wolff–Parkinson–White syndrome (with an associated delta wave)
➤ Pompe disease (with a wide QRS).

ASSESS THE QT INTERVAL

The QT interval is the time taken for ventricular depolarisation and repolarisation to occur. It is measured from the start of the Q wave to the end of the T wave. If no Q wave is present, you measure the QT from the start of the QRS complex.

It is difficult to give a reference range for the QT interval as it is heart rate dependent. In other words, the faster the patient's heart rate the quicker the ventricles must depolarise and repolarise. This results in a shorter QT value with faster heart rates. To overcome the problem of needing a separate QT reference range for each heart rate, we 'correct' the QT value for the heart rate. This is known as the corrected QT value, or QTc.

Calculate the QTc as follows.

1 First identify leads II and V5 on your 12-lead ECG. These leads are selected as they usually have the most obvious T waves.
2 Measure 3 to 5 QT values in these leads. Be careful not to include any U waves in your measurements. You will use the largest QT value that you obtain later.
3 Next calculate the RR interval. In paediatrics, sinus arrhythmia is often present and so the RR interval will vary. To overcome this, we calculate an average RR interval over 5 to 10 beats.
4 From the longest QT value and the average RR value (with both measured in seconds) you can now correct the QT using Bazett's formula:

$$QTc = \frac{QT}{\sqrt{R-R}}$$

We typically set a reference range of a QTc of less than 440 ms (0.44 seconds) as being normal. However, it is important to be aware that neonates typically have a slightly longer QTc when compared to older children and adults. Females also have a slightly longer QTc than males. A minority of people with long QT syndrome will have a QTc of less than 440 ms. Equally, a minority of normal people will have a QTc of greater than 440 ms. A QTc of over 480 ms is always considered abnormal in all groups.

The QTc is very important in paediatric practice and should be calculated each time a paediatric ECG is performed. The significance of the QTc and clinical problems are discussed as a separate entity in long QT syndrome (*see* pages 168–70).

FORMULATE A CONCLUSION

If you work through the ECG in a logical fashion, as described above, you will have all the information you need to form an opinion on the ECG; often this will result in the conclusion of a normal ECG for the age of the child. It is important to document your ECG findings in the notes, and file the ECG for future comparison. If in doubt, ask for help.

PAEDIATRIC ECG REFERENCE RANGES

Throughout this chapter we have alluded to the fact that the ECG morphology and normal values are age dependent. This can make interpretation difficult for the beginner. The appendix at the back of this book displays normal values for the paediatric ECG as reported across a wide range of literature. The ranges quoted are the 2nd to 98th centile for each age. It will be a useful tool when interpreting the ECG. As mentioned at the start of this chapter, knowing the age of the patient is vital before moving through any of these stages.

CHAPTER 5

Investigations for suspected cardiac disorders

Introduction
Electrocardiogram
Chest X-ray
Transthoracic echocardiogram
Transoesophageal echocardiogram
Ambulatory ECG recordings
Exercise testing
Diagnostic cardiac catheterisation
Cardiac MRI

INTRODUCTION

Unlike some areas of paediatrics, cardiology has a limited number of investigations. It is important to understand what each investigation is so that you can explain to parents what is involved. It is also important for you as a clinician to understand the indications, and limitations, of each test. Nothing can replace a detailed history and examination of the child.

Possible tests include:

➤ electrocardiogram
➤ chest X-ray (CXR)
➤ transthoracic echocardiogram (Echo)
➤ transoesophageal echocardiogram (TOE)
➤ ambulatory ECG recordings
➤ exercise testing
➤ diagnostic cardiac catheterisation
➤ cardiac magnetic resonance imaging (MRI).

This chapter gives a summary of the core investigations used in paediatric cardiology. Some of these are available only in tertiary cardiology centres; others are available in other settings such as general practice or A&E.

ELECTROCARDIOGRAM

The electrocardiogram is one of the first-line investigations in any suspected cardiovascular disease. It provides detailed information about both structure and function of the heart. ECGs are quick and easy to obtain, painless for the child and provide a good starting point for cardiovascular assessment.

A core skill of any paediatric trainee is to be able to record and interpret an ECG on children of all ages. Figure 5.1 demonstrates the exact location of the ECG lead placement to obtain a 12-lead ECG. Lead position is important to ensure that the interpretation is subsequently correct. Interpretation of the ECG in children is discussed in great detail in Chapter 4.

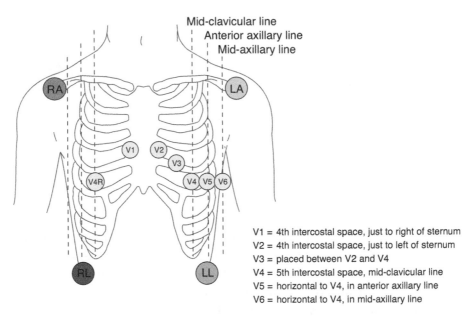

V1 = 4th intercostal space, just to right of sternum
V2 = 4th intercostal space, just to left of sternum
V3 = placed between V2 and V4
V4 = 5th intercostal space, mid-clavicular line
V5 = horizontal to V4, in anterior axillary line
V6 = horizontal to V4, in mid-axillary line

FIGURE 5.1 ECG lead-placement landmarks (with all leads on the left-hand side)

CHEST X-RAY

The chest X-ray is another frequently performed investigation early in the investigation of suspected structural cardiac disease. The CXR will provide some understanding of heart shape, size and position in the thorax. Some information can be obtained about pulmonary blood flow (based on the degree of pulmonary vascular markings). It is also useful in excluding lung pathology (e.g. pneumothorax, congenital pneumonia) in the neonate with low saturations, which may not be cardiac in nature.

Many cardiac defects will have a normal chest X-ray (e.g. mild aortic or pulmonary stenosis, small VSD, arrhythmias). The information obtained from a CXR should be combined with the ECG findings and clinical assessment.

Table 5.1 displays some of the possible findings on a chest X-ray that may suggest cardiac disease as a cause.

TABLE 5.1 CXR findings and their significance in cardiac disease

Chest X-ray findings	Possible cardiac causes
Apex in the right side of the chest (dextrocardia)	• Full body situs inversus • Atrial isomerism • Complex congenital heart disease • Mediastinal shift (e.g. pneumothorax)
Cardiomegaly	• Cardiomyopathy • Volume loaded heart (e.g. large VSD) • Pericardial effusion • Ebstein's anomaly ('wall to wall heart') • Ventricular hypertrophy
Plethoric lung fields (Increased pulmonary vascular markings)	• Left to right shunts (e.g. VSD, ASD) • Pulmonary oedema (e.g. cardiomyopathy)
Oligaemic lung fields (Reduced pulmonary vascular markings)	• Tetralogy of Fallot • Pulmonary atresia • Severe pulmonary stenosis • Ebstein's anomaly • PPHN
Narrow mediastinum ('Egg on side')	• Transposition of the great arteries
Upturned apex ('Boot-shaped heart')	• Tetralogy of Fallot • Pulmonary atresia • Right ventricular hypertrophy
Small heart with pulmonary venous congestion ('Snowman in a snowstorm')	• Total anomalous pulmonary venous drainage (TAPVD)
Rib notching	• Late sign of coarctation of the aorta
Absent thymic shadow	• 22q11 microdeletion/DiGeorge syndrome (associated with congenital heart defects)

TRANSTHORACIC ECHOCARDIOGRAM

A transthoracic echocardiogram is an ultrasound assessment of the heart. It is a dynamic process providing real-time information, but it is user dependent. It is vital in day-to-day paediatric cardiology, as it allows clear visualisation of all the anatomy discussed in Chapter 2. We can detect abnormal connections of blood vessels, narrowing of valves or septal defects, to name but a few. As children (especially neonates) have thin chest walls, clear and detailed images can often be obtained, allowing us to see details that may not always be possible in adults. Three-dimensional (3D) echo is now in use, especially in the pre-operative assessment to help plan corrective surgery for defects such as complete AVSD.

Echo does not always have to be used for structure; much information about cardiac function can be assessed in both systole and diastole, as discussed in the section Basic Cardiovascular Physiology in Chapter 2. Functional echo assessment is often used to guide inotropic and fluid resuscitation in the neonatal and paediatric intensive care units. Figure 5.2 displays some examples of static echo images obtained from a child with a normal heart.

FIGURE 5.2A–D A. Apical four-chamber view; **B.** Parasternal long axis view;

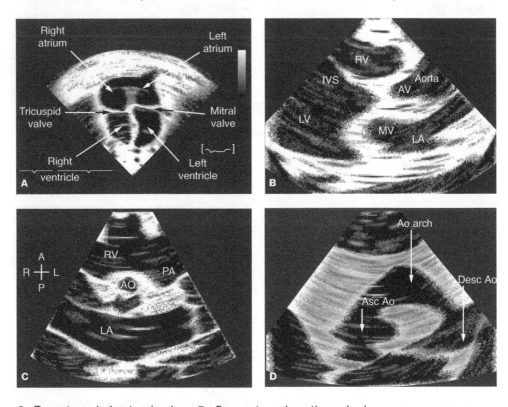

C. Parasternal short axis view; **D.** Suprasternal aortic arch view

Echo assessment is a huge and specialised subject that is out of the scope of this book, but many useful resources and training courses exist to learn this useful skill.

TRANSOESOPHAGEAL ECHOCARDIOGRAM

A transoesophageal echocardiogram is also an ultrasound assessment of the heart, but in a TOE the ultrasound probe views the heart from the posterior aspect by placing the probe down the oesophagus. The benefit of this method is that the ultrasound beam has less distance to travel towards the heart than the transthoracic echo, which has to traverse the chest wall.

As a result of this, TOE has some advantages over transthoracic echo, including:

➤ better visualisation of valves (important when considering a diagnosis of infective endocarditis)

➤ better visualisation of the atrial septum (important for diagnosing ASD)

➤ better visualisation of the pulmonary veins

➤ better for identifying intracardiac thrombus formation.

However, TOE requires a general anaesthesia in children, and usually sedation in adults. It is therefore not a practical test for routine use. In children, a good echocardiographer can obtain most of the information needed via a transthoracic echo. In those children who need further imaging, a TOE would then be used.

AMBULATORY ECG RECORDINGS

Ambulatory ECG devices (e.g. Holter monitor) are portable devices that are fixed to the child for a set period of time and provide constant ECG recordings in this time frame. They are typically attached for 24 hours, but can be kept on for up to 7 days, depending on the clinical situation.

The device is then downloaded and the traces can be reviewed. It is important that the child and their guardians keep a diary of activities and symptoms, so the ECG recordings can be matched up to activity. For instance, a 10-year-old boy whose heart rate increases to a sinus rhythm of 150 beats per minute while playing football is not significant, but it may be significant if that increase was sudden while asleep.

This investigation is commonly used in children under investigation for a suspected arrhythmia, or to monitor treatment of a proven arrhythmia. It can also be used in children with significant syncope but who have a normal resting 12-lead ECG.

A similar device known as an ECG event recorder (e.g. Cardiomemo) can be used for much longer, often up to one month. It is activated by pressing a button (if leads are attached to the chest) or by placing the device against the bare chest (if no leads used) when symptoms occur. This device is more useful in people with infrequent symptoms.

EXERCISE TESTING

Exercise testing is a technique in which the patient is placed on an exercise device, such as a treadmill or bicycle, and made to do increasing levels of activity. Monitoring occurs at baseline, during the exercise and in the cool-down phase after exercise has stopped. Protocols exist in how to grade exercise (e.g. Bruce Protocol).

The monitoring that occurs for this test includes:

➤ blood pressure
➤ heart rate
➤ oxygen saturations
➤ ECG rhythm strip (with periodic 12-lead ECGs)
➤ symptoms experienced by the patient (e.g. breathlessness, dizziness, palpitations, chest pain).

In some cases you can monitor pulmonary function and anaerobic exercise threshold levels, but this is not routine.

The exercise test is useful to:

➤ assess for exercise-induced arrhythmias
➤ assess for ischaemic changes (e.g. with Kawasaki disease or aortic stenosis)
➤ assess exercise tolerance in children with significant congenital heart disease
➤ assess the QT interval during exercise (for those children with exercise-induced syncope with a normal 12-lead ECG)
➤ provide reassurance to families that exercise is safe in children with exercise-related symptoms thought to be non-cardiac in nature.

In paediatrics, many of these tests have a doctor present along with the technical staff, in the rare event that a significant arrhythmia (e.g. ventricular tachycardia) does occur.

The important consideration for exercise testing in the paediatric population is the age of the child. Some children are too small, either physically or developmentally, to go on a bike/treadmill, and other ways of investigating may need to be considered.

DIAGNOSTIC CARDIAC CATHETERISATION

This is an invasive test, using a mix of contrast and X-ray to show cardiac structure, and pressure transducers to record intracardiac pressures and oxygen saturations. It requires the child to be under a general anaesthetic. Cardiac catheterisation is used less frequently for diagnostic purposes since the improvement in echocardiography and other imaging tools (such as MRI).

Indications for diagnostic cardiac catheterisation in children include the following.

➤ To describe complex anatomy when echocardiographic assessments are not clear (often in the case of multiple co-lateral blood vessels in the presence of major congenital heart disease).
➤ Assessment of the anatomy of the pulmonary blood vessels, and pulmonary vascular resistance, between staged surgical procedures for univentricular repair (e.g. Norwood procedure; *see* pages 146–9).
➤ To delineate coronary artery anatomy (e.g. in follow-up of Kawasaki disease with coronary artery aneurysms suspected).

➤ Assessment of pulmonary arterial hypertension.
➤ As part of an interventional catheter, to ensure the intervention is suitable and can be performed safely.

The majority of cardiac catheterisations performed in children are now interventional catheters. Examples of when they are used are included throughout Chapter 6.

CARDIAC MRI

Cardiac magnetic resonance imaging is an increasingly used imaging modality in the assessment of the cardiovascular system. It can be useful in delineating not only anatomy but cardiac function, especially of the right ventricle, an area in which traditional echocardiography is less effective. Cardiac MRI scans require the child to lie very still for a significant proportion of the time – as a result, many children require a general anaesthetic for this procedure. Cardiac MRI has a big role in adult congenital heart disease services, where it is harder for the echo assessment to see the same level of detail as in children.

Indications for cardiac MRI include the following.

➤ Additional diagnostic information in congenital heart disease.
➤ Assessment of cardiac function (especially the right ventricle).
➤ Follow-up after surgical correction of congenital heart disease, especially:
  ➢ coarctation of the aorta
  ➢ tetralogy of Fallot
  ➢ transposition of the great arteries.

As with any MRI, the usual contraindications apply. This is important as many people with congenital heart disease will have a pacemaker *in situ*. Older pacemakers are a contraindication for MRI. Many of the newer pacemakers are compatible with MRI scans. In order to be sure, check with the manufacturer of the pacemaker that the patient is using.

CHAPTER 6

A–Z of paediatric cardiac disorders and procedures

A

Acquired heart disease
Acyanotic congenital heart disease
Alagille syndrome – *see* Syndromes associated with cardiac
   abnormalities
Anomalous origin of left coronary artery from pulmonary artery
   (ALCAPA)
Aortic regurgitation (AR)
Aortic stenosis (AS)
Arrhythmias
Arterial switch procedure
Atrial septal defect (ASD)
Atrioventricular septal defect (AVSD)

ACQUIRED HEART DISEASE

Heart problems in the majority of children are congenital in nature; that is, the child is born with the problem.

However, a small proportion of children develop heart disease having been born with a normal heart. Although less common than congenital heart disease (CHD), it is important to appreciate.

Often, acquired heart disease in children follows an infection, inflammatory process or toxin exposure. Despite this, a cause is not always found for certain diseases.

Currently, the majority of heart disease in adults is acquired (e.g. ischaemic heart disease), but due to advances in paediatric cardiology, more people are growing up into adulthood with congenital heart disease.

The important paediatric acquired heart diseases include:

➤ Kawasaki disease
➤ cardiomyopathies
➤ pericarditis
➤ myocarditis
➤ infective endocarditis (although often with a background diagnosis of a congenital heart disease)
➤ rheumatic fever
➤ certain types of arrhythmia.

These diseases are discussed throughout this book.

ACYANOTIC CONGENITAL HEART DISEASE

Acyanotic congenital heart disease is a term used to describe congenital defects affecting the heart, but resulting in a pink child, with normal oxygen saturations. This is the opposite to cyanotic congenital heart disease (*see* page 97).

Acyanotic heart defects are the commonest type of congenital heart disease, accounting for 70% of all cases.

Examples of acyanotic congenital heart disease (in decreasing order of incidence) include:

➤ ventricular septal defects (VSD)
➤ atrial septal defects (ASD)
➤ patent ductus arteriosus (PDA)
➤ coarctation of the aorta
➤ pulmonary stenosis (PS)
➤ aortic stenosis (AS).

Acyanotic heart defects can range from asymptomatic minor defects through to symptoms of severe congestive heart failure requiring surgical and medical intervention.

The three main pathologies in the acyanotic heart disease group include the following.

1 High pulmonary blood flow and volume overload:
   ➤ left to right shunt (e.g. VSD, ASD, PDA)
   ➤ the high pulmonary blood flow makes the child breathless, but pink
   ➤ often do not present at birth, as high pulmonary vascular resistance (PVR) in the newborn reduces left to right flow
   ➤ as the PVR falls over the first few days/weeks, the degree of shunting increases and the child may become symptomatic or a new murmur audible.

2 Left ventricular outflow tract obstruction:
   ➤ results in reduced systemic blood flow (mild to severe)
   ➤ the symptoms will depend of the degree of obstruction; critical obstruction will reduce in cardiogenic shock
   ➤ includes aortic stenosis and coarctation of the aorta.
3 Right ventricular outflow tract obstruction:
   ➤ results in reduced pulmonary blood flow (mild to severe)
   ➤ these children are not cyanosed if this is an isolated defect, as oxygenation of the blood remains unaffected. However, with associated lesions (e.g. a VSD) there can be right to left shunting resulting in a cyanotic heart disease
   ➤ includes pulmonary stenosis.

ANOMALOUS ORIGIN OF LEFT CORONARY ARTERY FROM PULMONARY ARTERY (ALCAPA)

The left coronary artery usually arises as the first branch from the ascending aorta, from the left aortic sinus. Figure 6.1A shows the typical anatomy of the coronary arteries, but much variation in the normal condition does exist.

ALCAPA is a congenital heart defect where the left coronary artery arises from the pulmonary artery (Figure 6.1B).

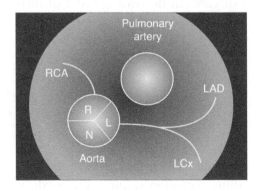 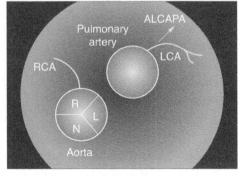

FIGURE 6.1A Normal coronary artery anatomy

FIGURE 6.1B The LCA arises from the PA (ALCAPA)

RCA – Right coronary artery; *LCA* – Left coronary artery; *LCx*– Circumflex artery (branch of LCA); *LAD* – Left anterior descending (branch of LCA); *PA* – Pulmonary artery.

ALCAPA is the most important coronary artery congenital defect in children, and it is usually an isolated defect. It is a rare, with an incidence of 1 in 300 000 live births.

The problem with ALCAPA is that the LCA arises from a vessel carrying deoxygenated blood and under relatively low pressure, and may even cause reversal of flow from the coronary artery to the PA. This means the myocardium supplied by the LCA is under significant risk of ischaemia and infarction.

ALCAPA typically presents with angina or myocardial infarction in infancy (see clinical features below).

➤ As the pulmonary vascular resistance falls in infancy less blood is provided to the left coronary artery, causing the angina/myocardial infarction. This can often be mistaken for gastro-oesophageal reflux or colic.

➤ Occasionally, an extensive collateral network of blood vessels around the myocardium can develop, allowing the child to be asymptomatic until older child/adulthood when they are at risk of sudden cardiac death or cardiomyopathy.

Treatment is with surgery to relocate the left coronary artery to its appropriate place along with medical management at the time of presentation and for any LV dysfunction.

Clinical features

Asymptomatic in first month

➤ Irritability
➤ Pallor } Usually after
➤ Sweating } feeding
➤ Congestive cardiac failure (*see* pages 84–6)
➤ Murmur of mitral regurgitation (due to damage of papillary muscles by infarction)
➤ Sudden cardiac death

Investigations

1 Cardiac enzymes (e.g. troponin T) may be elevated.
2 ECG can show a sinus tachycardia with evidence of ischaemia or infarction (ST segment changes in localised leads, usually anterolateral or deep Q waves).
3 CXR may show cardiomegaly.
4 Echo will demonstrate the LCA arising from the PA and mitral regurgitation and dilated or poor LV function.
5 Coronary angiography may be needed in some cases.

AORTIC REGURGITATION (AR)

Aortic regurgitation is the description of blood in the ascending aorta leaking (regurgitating) back through the aortic valve and into the left ventricle, during diastole, for a variety of reasons (Figure 6.2A, B).

AR itself is not a diagnosis. Causes of AR include:

➤ damaged aortic valve (e.g. post balloon valvuloplasty for aortic stenosis, post surgery)
➤ congenitally abnormal aortic valve (e.g. bicuspid aortic valve)
➤ aortic valve infective endocarditis
➤ dilatation of the aortic root (e.g. connective tissue diseases such as Marfan syndrome)

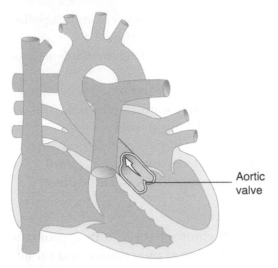

Aortic valve

FIGURE 6.2A The normal function of the aortic valve preventing backflow of blood into the left ventricle

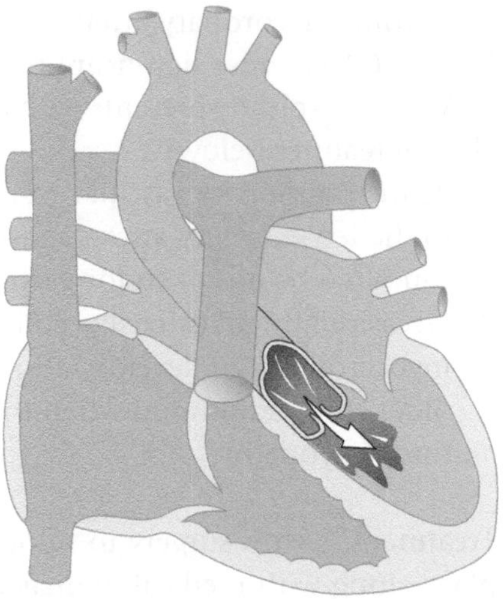

FIGURE 6.2B Aortic regurgitation, with failure of the aortic valve

➤ rheumatological diseases (e.g. vasculitis such as Kawasaki or Takayasu disease; systemic lupus erythematosus)
➤ systemic arterial hypertension
➤ rheumatic fever.

As with any disease of the valves, the severity can range from trivial to severe. This in turn will determine clinical features and subsequent management.

People with severe, acute onset AR (e.g. with dissection of dilated aorta) will present differently to those with chronic post-operative mild AR, for example.

Management of AR involves treating any underlying cause if possible, serial follow-up and then aortic valve replacement if severe. Medical treatments to reduce the afterload are possible.

Clinical features
> Asymptomatic
> Routine finding due to assessment for other condition (e.g. aortic root size in Marfan sysndrome)
> Shortness of breath
> Reduced exercise tolerance
> Fatigue
> Palpitations

Investigations
1 CXR is often normal, but can show mild cardiomegaly due to volume overload of the left ventricle. May show prominent aortic knuckle if dilated.
2 ECG can be normal, but may show left axis deviation for age.

(*continued*)

Clinical features

> Murmur
  ✓ Early diastolic murmur at aortic area
  ✓ Loudest at the start of diastole then gets quieter
  ✓ Loudest when patient sat forward and breath held at the end of expiration
> Collapsing pulse
> Displaced apex

Investigations

3 Echo will demonstrate the aortic regurgitation, along with the volume and function of the left ventricle. It may also help to identify the cause (e.g. dilated aortic root).

4 Further investigations should be guided by the suspected cause of the AR.

AORTIC STENOSIS (AS)

Aortic stenosis is a narrowing in the left ventricular outflow tract (LVOT), causing LVOT obstruction and increasing the workload on the left ventricle with potential left ventricular hypertrophy and dysfunction.

The spectrum of severity can range from mild through to critical aortic stenosis.

Critical aortic stenosis is defined as a narrowing in the LVOT of a neonate that causes an obstruction so severe that the systemic circulation is duct dependent.

The LVOT obstruction can occur at three main sites and can involve more than one level:

➤ subvalvular aortic stenosis
  ➣ this narrowing just below the aortic valve level at the exit of the left ventricle
  ➣ often associated with other defects (e.g. VSD, HOCM, interrupted aortic arch)
➤ valvular aortic stenosis
  ➣ often due to a congenitally abnormal aortic valve in children
  ➣ not usually associated with any major genetic defect
➤ supravalvular aortic stenosis
  ➣ this narrowing occurs above the aortic valve level, with a narrowing usually in the sinotubular junction of the ascending aorta
  ➣ associated with Williams syndrome.

The clinical features of aortic stenosis can vary dramatically depending on the age of the child, the severity of the obstruction, associated defects and the site of obstruction (see below).

Once again, management depends on lots of factors, mainly the severity and symptoms of the child.

➤ Commence prostaglandin treatment for critical aortic stenosis and arrange urgent transfer to a paediatric cardiac unit.
➤ Observation and serial follow-up is the commonest management for most cases.

➤ Aortic balloon valvuloplasty (dilating the obstruction with a balloon during cardiac catheter) is sometimes used in neonates and children.
➤ Aortic valve replacement or Ross Procedure (changing pulmonary valve to aortic valve position, with insertion of a donor tissue pulmonary valve).
➤ Surgical resection of the obstruction (especially if muscular obstruction to subvalvular area).

Clinical features

> Asymptomatic
> Chest pain (especially on exertion)
> Syncope (especially on exertion)
> Shortness of breath
> Murmur
  ✓ Ejection systolic murmur
  ✓ Loudest at upper right sternal edge
  ✓ Radiates to carotids
  ✓ Carotid or suprasternal thrill
> Altered pulse character
  ✓ Slow rising
  ✓ Reduced volume (absent in critical AS) Ejection click (with valvular AS)
> Quiet second heart sound
> Apical heave

Evidence of associated syndromes/defects may also be present

Investigations

1 ECG may demonstrate left ventricular dominance or hypertrophy.
2 CXR is usually normal, but may show mild cardiomegaly in long-term disease.
3 Exercise testing may show evidence of ischaemia (ST changes) during increasing exercise, along with fall in blood pressure.
4 Echo will demonstrate the area of narrowing, the morphology of the valve and any associated defects (e.g. VSD) or complications (e.g. LV hypertrophy or LV dysfunction).
5 Diagnostic catheter would show a high pressure gradient across the LVOT, but is usually only performed as part of a balloon valvuloplasty, as echo is very accurate.

ARRHYTHMIAS

Arrhythmia is a term used to describe any abnormal electrical pattern seen within the heart.

Arrhythmias are typically considered as tachycardia (i.e. heart rate over the upper limit of normal for age) or bradycardia (i.e. heart rate under the lower limit of normal for age).

Each arrhythmia has its own specific management and prognosis.

Childhood arrhythmias are a huge subject. This page is a very basic overview. Further arrhythmias are discussed in the SVT and VT pages in this chapter and throughout Chapter 4. For further details a more detailed paediatric arrhythmia book is recommended.

The flow chart below gives a basic outline of how arrhythmias in children can be classified, and some examples of each cause.

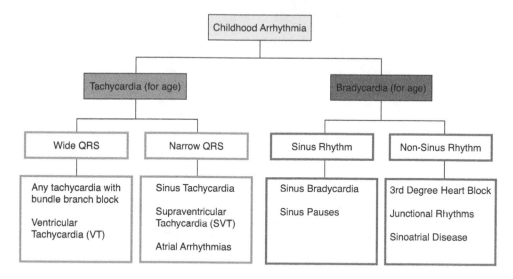

FIGURE 6.3 Childhood arrhythmias

ARTERIAL SWITCH PROCEDURE

This is a surgical operation used to correct transposition of the great arteries (TGA) (*see* page 195). It is now the main surgical treatment for TGA.

It is also less commonly referred to as the Jatene procedure.

It is a major neonatal cardiac surgical procedure.

The operation involves the following.

➤ The aorta and pulmonary artery are removed from their transposed positions.

➤ The aorta is sutured onto the old pulmonary artery root:
  ➢ pulmonary artery root → neo-aorta.

➤ The pulmonary artery is sutured onto the old aortic root.

➤ The coronary arteries are then removed from the original aortic root and re-implanted on the neo-aortic root.

➤ Any atrial septal damage from balloon septostomy (*see* page 171) is repaired, along with any other associated defects.

The stages of the procedure can be seen in Figure 6.4.

This operation is performed with cardiopulmonary bypass and involves a mid-line sternotomy incision.

It is usually performed in the first two weeks of life.

➤ In TGA the left ventricle supports the pulmonary circulation, which after the first few days is under lower pressure than the systemic circulation.

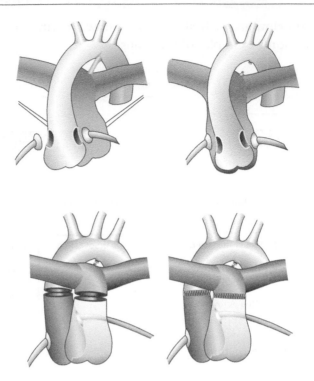

FIGURE 6.4 Arterial switch procedure

➤ If the LV is left attached to the pulmonary artery for too long, it adapts to supporting a lower pressure circulation.
➤ When the LV is reconnected to the aorta, it is then unable to support the systemic circulation and LV failure follows.

Careful follow up of these patients is needed for life. The following complications can occur in the long term:
➤ pulmonary stenosis
➤ damage to coronary arteries
➤ LV failure
➤ aortic valve insufficiency.

ATRIAL SEPTAL DEFECT (ASD)

The atrial septum is the wall that separates the left and right atria. Any communication between the two atria through the atrial septum is known as an atrial septal defect.

ASD is the third commonest congenital heart defect (comprising 7% of all congenital heart disease).

ASD is an example of acyanotic heart disease, and it can present at any age from neonate to adult, usually with an incidental murmur being noted by a healthcare professional or a stroke at an early age.

Different types of ASD are recognised:
➤ secundum ASD
➤ patent foramen ovale
➤ primum ASD (also known as a partial atrioventricular septal defect)
➤ sinus venosus ASD

ASDs are associated with:
➤ Holt–Oram syndrome
➤ Noonan syndrome
➤ Down syndrome
➤ Ellis–van Creveld syndrome.

Complications of ASD are often seen in older children and adults and include:
➤ high pulmonary blood flow and risk of pulmonary hypertension
➤ stroke
➤ thromboembolic risk
➤ arrhythmia risk (especially atrial flutter, atrial fibrillation and atrial tachycardia)
➤ association with migraine.

ASD closure is usually undertaken in the pre-school age (3–5 years old) to prevent complications, but can be closed at any age.

Secundum atrial septal defect

This is the commonest type of ASD.

There is a defect in the centre of the atrial septum allowing left to right flow between the atria (Figure 6.5). There can be more than one defect within the atrial septum.

There is no flap of tissue that is seen in a PFO (see below under PFO).

May spontaneously close over time, but less likely in large defects and older children/adults.

Management is either with device closure via interventional cardiac catheter or surgical closure if the device closure is not possible.

Patent foramen ovale (PFO)

The foramen ovale is a normal inter-atrial communication present in the fetus (discussed in detail under Fetal circulation, page 16).

The foramen ovale is present at birth in almost every neonate, and is therefore considered part of the normal neonatal findings on echocardiography.

The shunt between the atria is at the same site as the secundum ASD, but there is a 'flap valve' present in a foramen ovale that normally fuses with the atrial septum to cause closure. When the foramen ovale does not close, the defect is known as a patent foramen ovale (PFO) (Figure 6.6).

Management is either with device closure via interventional cardiac catheter or surgical closure if the device closure is not possible.

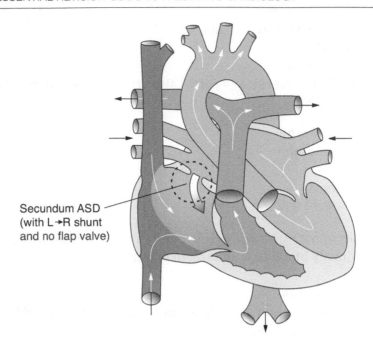

Secundum ASD
(with L→R shunt
and no flap valve)

FIGURE 6.5 The anatomy of a secundum atrial septal defect

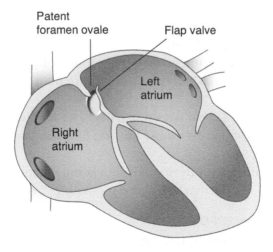

Patent
foramen ovale

Flap valve

Left
atrium

Right
atrium

FIGURE 6.6 The anatomy of a patent foramen ovale defect

Primum atrial septal defect

This defect is known as a partial atrioventricular septal defect, as it is very similar to an atrioventricular septal defect, but with no ventricular component.

It is discussed in more detail under Partial AVSD, page 77.

For comparison with other ASDs, the anatomy is displayed in Figure 6.7. Note that the ASD component is at the bottom of the atrial septum.

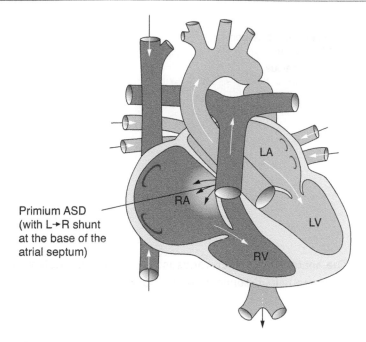

FIGURE 6.7 The anatomy of a primum atrial septal defect (or partial AVSD)

Sinus venosus ASD

A sinus venosus ASD involves a defect in the atrial septum at the junction of the superior vena cava (or less commonly the inferior vena cava) with the right atrium (Figure 6.8).

There is usually partial anomalous pulmonary venous drainage (PAPVD), often with the right upper pulmonary vein joining the superior vena cava (allowing left to right shunting).

This is the least common form of ASD.

Management of a sinus venosus ASD is with surgical correction only.

Clinical features

> Asymptomatic
> Found during cardiac assessment due to:
> > incidental murmur
> > known/suspected genetic syndrome
> > early thromboembolic event
> > severe migraines

Investigations

1 CXR can be normal. It may show cardiomegaly and increased pulmonary vascular markings due to left to right shunting, increasing pulmonary blood flow.

(*continued*)

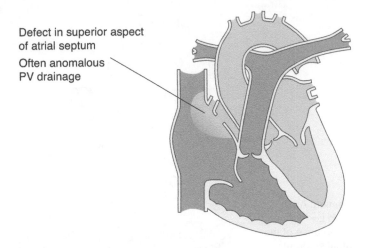

Defect in superior aspect of atrial septum

Often anomalous PV drainage

FIGURE 6.8 The anatomy of a sinus venosus defect (note the defect at the upper atrial septum with anomalous connection of a pulmonary vein)

Clinical features

> Features due to ASD tend not to present until adult life:
  > dyspnoea
  > palpitations
  > lethargy
  > heart failure
> Murmur
  ✓ Ejection systolic murmur
  ✓ Audible at the upper left sternal edge
  ✓ (NB: The murmur is not due to flow across the ASD; it is due to increased pulmonary blood flow)
> Fixed splitting of the second heart sound
> Dynamic praecordium due to increased right ventricular volume

Investigations

2 ECG can have some specific changes. It tends to be normal sinus rhythm, but can show atrial arrhythmias and evidence of pulmonary hypertension:
  > Secundum ASD
    ✓ right axis deviation
    ✓ partial or complete right bundle branch block
  > Primum ASD
    ✓ left axis deviation
    ✓ long PR interval
    ✓ partial or complete right bundle branch block
  > Sinus venosus ASD
    ✓ left axis deviation
    ✓ inverted P wave in lead III
    ✓ partial or complete right bundle branch block.
3 Echo will demonstrate the anatomy of the ASD and haemodynamic effects. Sometimes transoesophageal echo is needed to get clear views of the atrial septum (especially in older children and adults).

ATRIOVENTRICULAR SEPTAL DEFECT (AVSD)

Atrioventricular septal defect is a congenital heart disease that involves:

➤ one common atrioventricular valve (made up of five leaflets rather than a separate mitral and tricuspid valve)
➤ a defect in the atrial and ventricular septa.

AVSD accounts for 2% of all congenital heart defects (incidence 35 per 100 000 live births).

The range of AVSD is vast and depends on:

➤ the size of the atrial defect
➤ the size of the ventricular defect
➤ the size of both the ventricles (i.e. a balanced heart or unbalanced heart)
➤ the function of the common atrioventricular valve
➤ associated cardiac defects:
  ➢ coarctation of the aorta
  ➢ patent ductus arteriosus
  ➢ anomalous pulmonary venous drainage.

AVSD has a very strong association with Down syndrome, although it can occur as an isolated defect.

AVSD can be diagnosed in the antenatal period, but those that are not found often present with heart failure due to large shunting of blood from left to right (see below).

Management of all AVSD include the following.

➤ Manage associated heart failure (e.g. diuretics, ACE inhibitors).
➤ Maximise nutrition.
➤ Surgical repair around 3 to 6 months of life:
  ➢ a patch is used to close the ASD/VSD
  ➢ the five leaflet common valve is divided into two separate valves.
➤ Close follow-up – many children need a repair or replacement of one of the atrioventricular valves in later life.

Two main types of AVSD exist: complete and partial AVSD.

Complete atrioventricular septal defect (CAVSD)

This type of AVSD is associated with both atrial and ventricular septal defects with one common atrioventricular valve (Figure 6.9).

Partial atrioventricular septal defect

This is a form of AVSD with an atrial component in the lower portion of the atrial septum and abnormalities of the left atrioventricular valve. But there is no ventricular septal defect component. There are two separate ventricular openings (Figure 6.10).

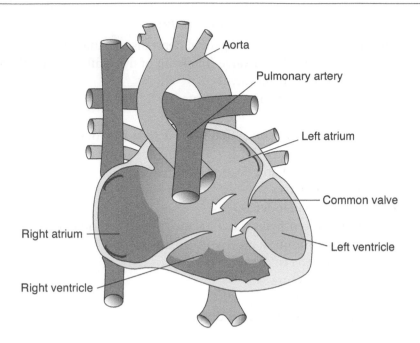

FIGURE 6.9 Complete atrioventricular septal defect

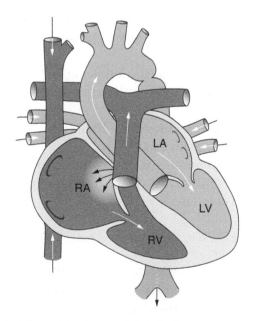

FIGURE 6.10 Partial atrioventricular septal defect

Partial AVSD is also known as a primum atrial septal defect, but it is important to remember that there is an abnormal left atrioventricular valve.

Figure 6.11 summarises the difference between the partial and complete AVSD types.

Partial AVSD   Complete AVSD

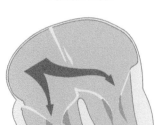 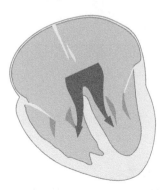

FIGURE 6.11 Comparison of the anatomy of partial and complete AVSD

Clinical features

> Antenatal diagnosis
> Asymptomatic (usually partial AVSD)
> Found due to cardiac assessment as routine part of Down syndrome investigation
> Present in first weeks of life with heart failure
> Recurrent lower respiratory tract infections
> Failure to thrive
> Poor feeding/sweating with feeds
> Respiratory distress
> Tachycardia
> Hepatomegaly
> Murmur (may be quiet or absent if large holes and little pressure gradient)
> Dynamic praecordium due to increased right ventricular volume
> Clinical features of Down syndrome

Investigations

1 CXR can be normal. It may show cardiomegaly and increased pulmonary vascular markings due to left to right shunting, increasing pulmonary blood flow.
2 ECG tends to be normal sinus rhythm. It can show evidence of pulmonary hypertension.
> Complete AVSD
   ✓ superior axis deviation
   ✓ partial or complete right bundle branch block
   ✓ long PR interval
> Partial AVSD (Primum ASD)
   ✓ left axis deviation
   ✓ long PR interval
   ✓ partial or complete right bundle branch block.
3 Echo will demonstrate the anatomy of the AVSD, haemodynamic effects and associated lesions.
4 Consider karyotyping for Down syndrome.

> Berlin Heart
> Bicuspid aortic valve
> Blalock–Taussig (BT) shunt

BERLIN HEART

The Berlin Heart is a specialised device which acts as an artificial heart until a suitable donor for cardiac transplant can be found, or on rare occasions until spontaneous recovery occurs.

It is only performed in two UK centres for children (Freeman Hospital, Newcastle & Great Ormond Street Hospital, London).

The Berlin Heart is also known as a ventricular assist device (VAD). Depending on the clinical situation this can support either:

➤ both ventricles, known as a biventricular assist device or BiVAD (Figure 6.12A)

➤ just the left ventricle, known as a left ventricular assist device, or LVAD (Figure 6.12B).

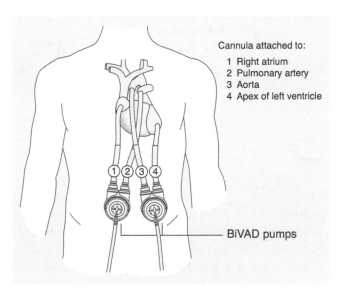

Cannula attached to:
1 Right atrium
2 Pulmonary artery
3 Aorta
4 Apex of left ventricle

BiVAD pumps

FIGURE 6.12A Biventricular assist device (BiVAD)

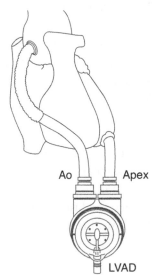

Ao   Apex

LVAD

FIGURE 6.12B Left ventricular assist device (LVAD)

The Berlin Heart has one tube coming out of the ventricle draining the blood. An external chamber collects the blood and then pumps it back to the heart via a second tube going to the exit vessel of this ventricle. This is a single system in LVAD and is duplicated in BiVAD, as demonstrated above. The pump therefore acts as the heart, irrespective of how poor the ventricular function is.

The Berlin Heart allows the child to be awake with a degree of mobility. It therefore has advantages over extracorporeal membrane oxygenation (ECMO). The Berlin Heart does not help with respiratory function (e.g. oxygenation).

The main indication for using the Berlin Heart is pre-cardiac transplant (e.g. with cardiomyopathy, or severe heart failure in single ventricle systems).

The Berlin Heart is not without complications. There is a risk of thromboembolic events if clots form in the VAD pumping chamber. Anticoagulation is very important in these children.

BICUSPID AORTIC VALVE

The aortic valve should normally be made up of three leaflets (Figure 6.13A).

In around 1%–2% of the population the aortic valve is composed of only two leaflets (more common in males and in those with a positive family history of bicuspid aortic valve).

➤ 'True' bicuspid aortic valve:
  ➢ complete absence of one of the commissures (point where the valve leaflets meet), resulting in only two leaflets of the valve
  ➢ this is shown in Figure 6.13B.
➤ 'Functional' bicuspid aortic valve:
  ➢ fusion of two valve leaflets together, but all three leaflets still identifiable
  ➢ this is shown in Figure 6.13C.

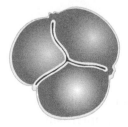 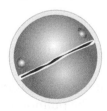 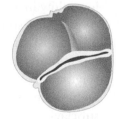

FIGURE 6.13A Normal trileaflet aortic valve

FIGURE 6.13B True bicuspid aortic valve with only two leaflets visible

FIGURE 6.13C Functional bicuspid aortic valve with fusion of two of the leaflets but all three still visible

The bicuspid aortic valve is associated with other congenital heart defects in children, and although bicuspid aortic valves are usually isolated it is important to exclude these defects. Common associations include:

➤ coarctation of the aorta (30% of children with coarctation have a bicuspid aortic valve)
➤ interrupted aortic arch
➤ hypoplastic left heart syndrome.

The natural progression of bicuspid aortic valve is variable.
➤ The majority function for a lifetime with no complications.
➤ Some develop valvular aortic stenosis (especially with increasing age).
➤ A few can develop aortic regurgitation.
➤ Risk of dilatation of the ascending aorta.

Management of a bicuspid aortic valve tends to involve serial echo assessments to monitor the natural history as described above. Treatment of associated conditions takes precedent. Occasionally, aortic valve replacement needs to occur, or balloon valvuloplasty.

Clinical features

> Asymptomatic
> Routine finding due to assessment for other condition (e.g. coarctation of aorta)
> May have signs of mild aortic stenosis, including murmur

Investigations

1 CXR and ECG are usually normal.
2 Echo will demonstrate the bicuspid aortic valve and assess for any stenosis or regurgitation. Echo will also identify associated cardiac defects.

BLALOCK–TAUSSIG (BT) SHUNT

The Blalock–Taussig shunt is a surgical procedure that is used to increase pulmonary blood flow in a cyanotic congenital heart defect.

Two types of BT shunt exist:
1 Traditional BT shunt
   ➤ The subclavian artery is directly attached to the pulmonary artery (Figure 6.14).
   ➤ As blood passes around the aorta, a proportion will pass down the subclavian artery and into the pulmonary arteries, thus increasing pulmonary blood flow.
   ➤ The problem is reduced blood supply to the affected arm, which can cause a discrepancy in size of the arms as the child grows (and clinically an absent brachial pulse in that arm).
2 Modified BT shunt
   ➤ This is the newer and more commonly used technique.
   ➤ A synthetic tube is connected between the subclavian artery and the pulmonary artery (Figure 6.15).

➤ As blood passes around the aorta now, blood will pass down the subclavian artery to supply the arm and a proportion will pass down the modified BT shunt to the pulmonary circulation.
➤ The child will still have an intact pulse in the arm.

A
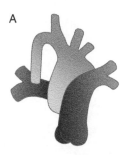

B
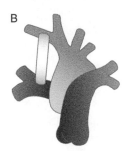

FIGURE 6.14 Traditional BT shunt   **FIGURE 6.15** Modified BT shunt

A BT shunt is a palliative operation to increase pulmonary blood flow and improve oxygen saturations until the child is old enough to grow for corrective or more palliative surgery. The child will still by cyanotic at the end of the shunt.

The risks of inserting a BT shunt are higher with the smaller weight of the child (especially less than 2 kg).

The BT shunt is usually inserted through a left or right lateral thoracotomy incision and does *not* involve going on cardiac bypass.

Potential situations when pulmonary blood flow is low and so a BT shunt may be used include:
➤ part of Stage I Norwood procedure for hypoplastic left heart syndrome
➤ pulmonary atresia
➤ critical pulmonary stenosis
➤ tetralogy of Fallot
➤ tricuspid atresia.

Cardiac catheterisation – *see* Chapter 5
Cardiac failure
Cardiomyopathy
Cardiopulmonary bypass surgery (CPB)
Cardioversion
CHARGE – *see* Syndromes associated with cardiac abnormalities
Coarctation of the aorta
Congenital heart disease (CHD)
Cyanotic congenital heart disease

CARDIAC FAILURE

Heart (cardiac) failure is a term used to describe the situation when the cardiac output fails to meet the demands of the child.

It is a condition usually associated with adult elderly care medicine; it also occurs in children.

Heart failure is a collective group of symptoms (see below). It is therefore *not* a diagnosis, and close evaluation of the child must be undertaken to find a cause for the heart failure.

Heart failure can often be misdiagnosed as a viral respiratory tract infection, especially in the winter months when bronchiolitis is common.

Causes of paediatric heart failure can be seen below (Table 6.1).

TABLE 6.1 Causes of paediatric heart failure

Category of heart failure	Examples
Pressure overload (obstructive lesions)	• Closure of duct in a duct-dependent lesion
	• Coarctation of the aorta
	• Aortic stenosis
	• Hypertension
Volume overload	• Large VSD
	• AVSD
	• PDA
Diseases of the myocardium	• Myocarditis
	• Cardiomyopathy
	• Myocardial ischaemia (e.g. ALCAPA)

(continued)

Category of heart failure	Examples
Arrhythmias	• SVT
	• VT
	• Incessant tachycardias
Non-cardiac related	• Sepsis
	• Severe anaemia

Treatment of heart failure in children is similar to that in adults.
➤ Treat the underlying cause.
➤ Careful fluid balance.
➤ Careful observations (e.g. regular blood pressure and heart rate).
➤ Reduce the pre-load:
  ➢ use diuretics
  ➢ e.g. furosemide, chlorothiazide, spironolactone.
➤ Increase cardiac contractility:
  ➢ give inotropes
  ➢ e.g. dopamine, dobutamine, milrinone, digoxin.
➤ Reduce the afterload:
  ➢ use ACE inhibitors
  ➢ e.g. captopril, enalapril.
➤ Evidence that β-blockers are beneficial (e.g. carvedilol).
➤ Consider:
  ➢ cardiac transplantation
  ➢ mechanical support (e.g. ECMO, Berlin Heart)
  ➢ biventricular pacing.

Clinical features

❯ Failure to thrive
❯ Poor feeding
❯ Short of breath
❯ Sweating on feeding
❯ Irritability/fatigue
❯ Reduced exercise tolerance
❯ Noisy breathing/coughing
❯ Older children may have typical adult signs (e.g. orthopnea, paroxysmal nocturnal dyspnoea)
❯ Pallor
❯ Tachycardia
❯ Tachypnoea

Investigations

1 Full blood count (FBC) is important to rule out anaemia.
2 Urea & electrolytes (U&E)/LFT to assess for end organ damage from hypoperfusion, but also in preparation for starting drugs that may affect renal function (e.g. ACE inhibitors).
3 Cardiomyopathy screen (*see* page 89) if indicated.
4 Investigations for myocarditis (*see* page 145) if indicated.

(*continued*)

Clinical features

> Wheeze
> Normal or low saturations
> Poor perfusion/cardiogenic shock
> Cardiomegaly (displaced apex beat)
> Hepatomegaly
> Gallop rhythm (HS I + II + III)
> Murmur may be present (often from mitral regurgitation)
> Ascites, pleural effusions and pedal oedema may also be present, again depending on the age of the child
> Clinical features of the underlying cause may also be found (e.g. absent femoral pulses)

Investigations

5 Blood gas (including lactate) is useful to assess for significant hypoperfusion.
6 ECG may show a sinus tachycardia. It may also give clues to the underlying cause of the heart failure (e.g. arrhythmia).
7 CXR may show cardiomegaly, pulmonary oedema and pulmonary venous congestion.
8 Echo will demonstrate any structural abnormalities. It will also allow you to assess the ventricular function and monitor treatment.

CARDIOMYOPATHY

Cardiomyopathy is a disease of the myocardium resulting in a degree of cardiac dysfunction and heart failure.

Cardiomyopathy can be divided into two main groups:

➤ primary cardiomyopathy – the disease is confined to the cardiac muscle only
➤ secondary cardiomyopathy – the disease of the myocardium is part of a generalised systemic disorder.

Cardiomyopathy is not common in the overall population, but it is more common in infants and younger children:

➤ 1.13 per 100 000 children under 18 years old
➤ 1.24 per 100 000 children under 10 years old.

There is often a genetic element to many cardiomyopathies; a detailed family history is vital.

The heart failure with cardiomyopathy is often mistaken for respiratory disorders in the first instance. It is important that if the child does not respond as expected to respiratory management a chest X-ray is performed and assessment of the heart size (cardiothoracic ratio) is made.

The clinical features of cardiomyopathy can range from an asymptomatic child to a child with severe heart failure (*see* page 84 and below).

When a child is diagnosed with a cardiomyopathy, a full cardiomyopathy screen must be undertaken (see investigations below). Identifying a cause of the cardiomyopathy will help guide treatment, prognosis and help screening for the remainder of the family. The list given is a guide; some tests may not be needed and others required. Consult local guidelines.

Management of cardiomyopathy will depend on the type, underlying cause and severity of the disease. General considerations include the following
➤ Treat/manage the underlying cause.
➤ Manage as heart failure (*see* page 84):
  ➣ diuretics
  ➣ ACE inhibitors
  ➣ β-blockers.
➤ Fluid restriction with close monitoring of fluid balance.
➤ Inotropic support (often with dobutamine and/or milrinone).
➤ May require ventilation.
➤ Rapid treatment of any arrhythmias (as will cause the child to decompensate rapidly).
➤ Insertion of pacemaker or implantable cardioverter defibrillators (as these children at high risk of sudden cardiac death).
➤ Mechanical support (either waiting for recovery of cardiac function or transplantation):
  ➣ ECMO (*see* page 106)
  ➣ Berlin Heart (*see* page 80).
➤ Surgical interventions include:
  ➣ treatment of congenital heart defects (e.g. ALCPA)
  ➣ myomectomy (removal of muscle obstructing the outflow tract in hypertrophic obstructive cardiomyopathy (HOCM))
  ➣ cardiac transplantation.
➤ Screen the family and have close discussion with genetics team.

Prognosis of cardiomyopathies is variable. Neonatal cardiomyopathy, or cardiomyopathy secondary to certain pathologies (e.g. inborn error of metabolism, neuromuscular disease), have a worse prognosis.

Cardiomyopathies are often described in more specific terms, based on the phenotypical appearance of the heart on echocardiogram. The three most encountered types in paediatric practice are briefly discussed below.

Dilated cardiomyopathy (DCM)
This is when the left ventricle (or occasionally both ventricles) is dilated, with impairment of contraction.

It is the commonest form or cardiomyopathy in children and usually presents under one year of age (0.57 per 100 000 children aged under 18 years *but* → 4.4 per 100 000 children aged less than 1 year).

The main causes of DCM are shown in Table 6.2.

TABLE 6.2 Major causes of dilated cardiomyopathy

Major group	Main examples
Idiopathic	
Myocarditis (*see* page 143)	
Neuromuscular disease	Duchenne muscular dystrophy
	Becker's muscular dystrophy
	Myotonic dystrophy
Familial (genetic)	
Arrhythmia	Recurrent or persistent tachycardia
Inborn errors of metabolism	Glycogen storage diseases
	Mucopolysaccharidoses
	Fatty acid oxidation defects
Nutritional deficiency	Vitamin B deficiency
	Vitamin D deficiency
Toxin related	Post-chemotherapy (especially with anthracyclines) Iron overload
Coronary artery disease	ALCAPA (*see* page 66)
	Myocardial infarction

Hypertrophic cardiomyopathy (HCM)

This is when the myocardium is hypertrophied without a structural heart defect.

It is the second commonest form of paediatric cardiomyopathy (0.2% of the population).

It is important as it can cause sudden cardiac death in children/young adults.

If the LV becomes so hypertrophied that it obstructs the left ventricular outflow tract, the disease is known as hypertrophic obstructive cardiomyopathy (HOCM).

The causes of HCM are shown in Table 6.3.

TABLE 6.3 Major causes of hypertrophic cardiomyopathy

Major group	Main examples
Idiopathic	
Familial	(often autosomal dominant inheritance)
Syndromic diseases	Noonan syndrome (*see* page 183)
	Leopard syndrome (*see* page 183)
Inborn errors of metabolism	Pompe disease (glycogen storage disease: acid maltase deficiency)
	Danon disease (glycogen storage disease: lysosome protein deficiency)
	Fabry disease (lysosomal storage disease: α-galactosidase A deficiency)
Mitochondrial disorders	Friedreich's ataxia (spinocerebellar degeneration)

Restrictive cardiomyopathy

This disease is associated with abnormal compliance of the ventricle wall, resulting in abnormal ventricular filling (i.e. a disease of diastolic impairment).

The ventricle is often stiff and rigid, making ventricular filling during diastole difficult.

Although less common than HCM and DCM, it is important as it carries a very high mortality in children.

The treatment of choice is heart transplantation.

The causes of restrictive cardiomyopathy are shown in Table 6.4.

TABLE 6.4 Causes of restrictive cardiomyopathy

Major group	Main examples
Idiopathic	
Infiltrative disease	Haemochromatosis and iron overload
	Hypereosinophilia
Toxin related	Radiotherapy
	Post-chemotherapy (especially with anthracyclines)
Inborn errors of metabolism	Fabry disease (lysosomal storage disease: α-galactosidase A deficiency)
	Glycogen storage diseases
	Hurler syndrome (Type I mucopolysaccharidoses) Gaucher's disease (lysosomal storage disease)

Clinical features

> Asymptomatic
> Detected on screening (e.g. family history)
> Clinical features of heart failure (*see* page 85)
> Clinical features of any underlying syndrome or metabolic disease
> Sudden cardiac death
> Arrhythmias

Investigations

1 ECG may demonstrate hypertrophy or tachycardia but often displays non-specific changes that are not normal.
2 CXR is may show cardiomegaly and pulmonary oedema.
3 Echo will demonstrate the phenotype of the cardiomyopathy, allow functional assessment and rule out structural defects.
4 Cardiomyopathy screen often includes blood investigations for:
  a. FBC and blood film for vacuolated lymphocytes
  b. U&E/LFT/C reactive protein (CRP)/ erythrocyte sedimentation rate (ESR)/ Bone profile
  c. Serial viral titres

(*continued*)

Clinical features

> Murmur
  - ✓ May be due to mitral regurgitation associated with LV dilatation
  - ✓ May be similar to aortic stenosis, due to the LV outflow tract obstruction in HOCM

Investigations

d. Thyroid stimulating hormone (TSH) and free T_4
e. Carnitine
f. Ferritin and transferrin
g. Vitamin D, parathyroid hormone (PTH) and calcium
h. Vitamin B_1 (thiamine) and B_{12}
i. Folate
j. Blood gas
k. Lactate
l. Intermediary metabolites (e.g. pyruvate)
m. Serum amino acids
n. Non-esterified fatty acids
o. HIV serology
p. Glucose and insulin
q. Genetic screening (as indicated).
5 Cardiomyopathy screen often includes urine investigations for:
  a. Urinary amino acids
  b. Glycosaminoglycans
  c. Organic acids
  d. Oligosaccharides.

CARDIOPULMONARY BYPASS SURGERY (CPB)

Cardiopulmonary bypass surgery is a surgical technique that allows a machine and circuit to act as the heart (a pump) and the lungs (an oxygenator and carbon dioxide remover) during cardiac surgery.

This technique allows the heart to stop beating, and minimises the blood obstructing the surgeon's view of the heart.

CPB is usually carried out in cardiothoracic theatres for surgery. However, ECMO used in some PICUs is a form of CBP (*see* page 90).

A CPB circuit is shown in Figure 6.16. Blood leaves the circulation from a cannula placed in the venous system (e.g. femoral vein, vena cava or right atrium). It passes through an oxygenator where oxygen is added to the blood. It is then warmed and pumped back into the circulation via a cannula placed in the arterial system (e.g. ascending aorta).

Children that have cardiac surgery performed under CPB will often have two types of scars:

1 Midline sternotomy scar
2 Chest and mediastinal drain scars (often smaller scars in the subcostal region; can be more noticeable than the sternotomy scar).

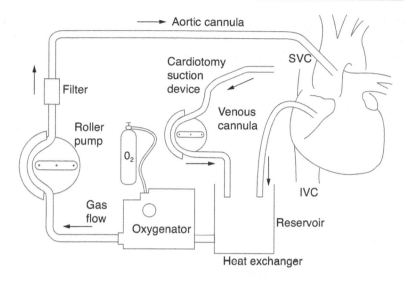

FIGURE 6.16 A simplified cardiopulmonary bypass circuit

CPB is generally needed in any child having an operation directly inside the heart or on the great vessels, or having a central shunt insertion.

Operations performed in children with CPB include:

➤ arterial switch procedure
➤ Norwood procedure
➤ Glenn shunt
➤ Fontan procedure
➤ tetralogy of Fallot repair
➤ complete AVSD repair
➤ and many more . . .

Not all cardiac surgery needs CPB. Non-bypass surgery includes:

➤ BT shunt
➤ repair of coarctation of the aorta
➤ pulmonary artery (PA) band
➤ ligation of PDA.

CARDIOVERSION

Cardioversion is a term used to describe the process of changing a patient's abnormal electrical cardiac rhythm back to a normal sinus rhythm.

Two main types of cardioversion exist:

➤ pharmacological (drug) cardioversion
➤ electrical (direct current (DC)) cardioversion.

Cardioversion can be carried out electively in people with stable arrhythmias or as an emergency procedure in haemodynamically significant arrhythmias.

To help with diagnosis, follow-up and future management of children with arrhythmias a 12-lead ECG should be recorded before, during (if possible) and after cardioversion. A rhythm strip is the minimal requirement that should be printed out, but this lacks a lot of the detail that a 12-lead ECG offers.

Pharmacological (drug) cardioversion

This method involves giving a drug that either rapidly or over time converts the heart back into a sinus rhythm.

Drugs sometimes used in cardioversion include:

➤ adenosine
➤ amiodarone
➤ flecainide
➤ lidocaine.

Good vascular access is needed for many of these drugs, sometimes via a central line (e.g. amiodarone).

If time allows, you should always seek advice from a paediatric cardiologist before attempting cardioversion of many rhythms.

Electrical (DC) cardioversion

This involves using a direct current from the defibrillator to deliver an electric current to 'reset' the heart into a sinus rhythm.

DC cardioversion can be of two types:

1 Asynchronous
  ➤ This is when the shock is delivered at any point in the cardiac cycle.
  ➤ Used in cardiac arrest at a dose of 4 J/kg in children.
  ➤ Used in arrhythmias where the defibrillator fails to deliver a synchronous shock, at a dose of 1 J/kg for the first shock and then 2 J/kg for each subsequent shock.
2 Synchronous
  ➤ This is when the shock is only delivered at the timing of the R wave of the QRS complex.
  ➤ This is beneficial as it means the shock is not delivered in the relative refractory period when the heart is at its most vulnerable and risk of inducing VF is therefore lower.
  ➤ Each defibrillator has a 'sync' setting to allow this to happen, but sometimes the defibrillator is unable to identify an R wave (seen with VT) and will not release its charge. You need to then resort to asynchronous cardioversion at this point.
  ➤ Used in arrhythmias (e.g. SVT, VT) when the child still has a pulse but has haemodynamic compromise.
  ➤ Used in arrhythmias at a dose of 1 J/kg for the first shock and then 2 J/kg for each subsequent shock.

➤ The child ideally needs to be sedated or anaesthetised prior to synchronised DC cardioversion.

COARCTATION OF THE AORTA

This is a narrowing in the aorta, usually the descending aorta (Figure 6.17).

Coarctation of the aorta is a form of left ventricular outflow tract obstruction. It may occur as an isolated defect, but is can be associated with:

➤ bicuspid aortic valve
➤ ventricular septal defects
➤ patent ductus arteriosus
➤ hypoplastic left heart syndrome.

It is more common in Turner syndrome (45XO karyotype).

The severity of the obstruction can range from mild (found as an incidental finding) through to a duct-dependent circulation in a neonate (presenting with cardiogenic shock as the duct closes).

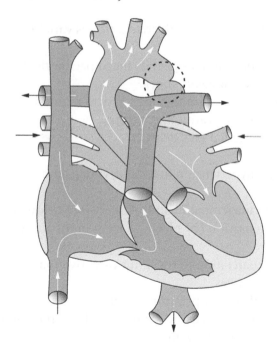

FIGURE 6.17 Coarctation of the aorta

There are two types of coarctation of the aorta. Understanding the differences between the two is important, as they present in different ways.

1 Pre-ductal coarctation
  ➤ 'Infant type'.
  ➤ The coarctation tends to be proximal or at the site of the ductus arteriosus insertion.

➤ The duct allows blood to bypass the obstruction.
➤ When the duct closes insufficient blood can get past the narrowing, causing a reduced cardiac output and systemic hypoperfusion.
➤ Tends to present with heart failure due to LV obstruction or duct-dependent cardiogenic shock.

2 Post-ductal coarctation
➤ 'Adult type' coarctation (although it can be found in children as well).
➤ The coarctation tends to be just distal to the site of the ductus arteriosus insertion.
➤ The presence of the duct does not matter, as it does not bypass the narrow segment of the aorta.
➤ Collateral blood vessels form over time to bypass the coarctation site. This is not a rapid process.
➤ Tend to present with young onset hypertension, possibly due to renal hypoperfusion causing activation of the rennin-angiotensin-aldosterone system.

The management of the patient with coarctation is variable.
➤ Pre-ductal
  ➢ Often need stabilisation as per advanced paediatric life support (APLS) guidelines if in cardiogenic shock.
  ➢ Commence prostaglandin therapy to try to maintain duct patency.
  ➢ Transfer to paediatric cardiology centre.
  ➢ Surgical repair needed (see below).
➤ Post-ductal
  ➢ Avoid treating hypertension in a child/young adult until coarctation is excluded.
  ➢ Options for management include surgery (see below) or interventional cardiac catheterisation (by placing a stent in the narrow segment).

Surgical options in coarctation of the aorta vary. Two main operations exist:
1 End-to-end anastomosis
➤ Most commonly used operation currently.
➤ Involves resecting the narrow segment of the aorta, and then joining the two ends back together again.
➤ Non-bypass operation, performed via a lateral thoracotomy.
2 Subclavian flap repair
➤ The left subclavian artery is disconnected from the upper limb, and used to widen the aorta at the site of narrowing.
➤ As a result there is a reduced/absent brachial pulse in the left upper limb.
➤ Long term there can be asymmetrical limb growth with this procedure.

Post-operative hypertension is a common complication, and responds to short-term antihypertensive therapy (e.g. with β-blockers). Always check BP in the right arm.

Follow-up of these children after repair is important as there is a risk of re-coarctation at the site of surgery needing further intervention (e.g. stent insertion). MRI is often used to monitor the aorta.

Clinical features

Pre-ductal coarctation
› Poor feeding
› Sudden collapse
› Tachypnoea/tachycardia
› Poor perfusion
› Absent femoral pulses
› Hypotension (may have upper limb BP higher than lower limb BP discrepancy)
› Hepatomegaly
› Murmur
  ✓ Maybe absent
  ✓ Systolic murmur
  ✓ Loudest at the back under left scapula
  ✓ May have pre- and post-ductal saturation discrepancy

Post-ductal coarctation
› Headaches or intracranial bleeds
› Chest pains or lower limb pains
› Fatigue
› Hypertension (upper limb BP higher than lower limb BP discrepancy)
› Weak femoral pulses
› Radio or brachiofemoral delay
› Murmur
  ✓ Systolic murmur
  ✓ Loudest at the back under left scapula
  ✓ Evidence of complications of hypertension (*see* page 119)

Investigations

Pre-ductal coarctation
1 CXR may show cardiomegaly and pulmonary oedema.
2 ECG is often normal, showing only a sinus tachycardia.
3 Echo will demonstrate the coarctation and other associated defects. Importance should be paid to the presence of the PDA. It will also help assess cardiac function.
4 Blood gasses/U&E/LFT.

Post-ductal coarctation
1 CXR may show cardiomegaly (due to left ventricular hypertrophy (LVH)) with rib notching (late sign of collateral vessel formation).
2 ECG may show LVH and possibly LV strain.
3 Echo will demonstrate the coarctation, but is much harder to see in older children and adults than in neonates.
4 MRI or cardiac catheterisation may be used as a diagnostic tool or for long-term follow-up.

CONGENITAL HEART DISEASE (CHD)

Congenital heart disease in children is the commonest group of congenital defects.

The reported incidence is 8 to 10 per 1000 live births (i.e. 0.8% to 1% of all live births). However, the incidence would be much higher if all terminations of pregnancy, still births or miscarriages were taken into account.

The spectrum of severity of CHD is huge, ranging from the tiny ventricular septal defect of no consequence through to single ventricle systems and duct-dependent circulations.

Congenital heart disease is divided into:
➤ acyanotic CHD (*see* page 65)
➤ cyanotic CHD (*see* page 97).

The frequency of individual defect varies. Table 6.5 displays the commonest forms of congenital heart disease, although it is difficult to clarify numbers, as many minor defects are never detected.

TABLE 6.5 Common congenital heart defects

Defect	% of all congenital heart disease
Ventricular septal defect (VSD)	30
Patent ductus arteriosus (PDA)	12
Atrial septal defect (ASD)	7
Pulmonary stenosis (PS)	7
Aortic stenosis (AS)	5
Coarctation of the aorta	5
Tetralogy of Fallot (ToF)	5
Transposition of the great arteries (TGA)	5
Atrioventricular septal defects (AVSD)	2
Bicuspid aortic valve	1

Risk factors for having a baby born with congenital heart disease have been difficult to prove, but do include:
➤ a positive family history in a first degree relative only
➤ known genetic syndrome in the baby (e.g. trisomy 21, 22q11 microdeletion)
➤ other anomalies present in the baby
➤ maternal illness pre-pregnancy:
  ➢ diabetes – especially transposition of the great arteries, truncus arteriosus and tricuspid atresia
  ➢ systemic lupus erythematosus – risk of congenital heart block
  ➢ phenylketonuria – especially tetralogy of Fallot, coarctation of the aorta and hypoplastic left heart syndrome
➤ maternal illness during pregnancy
  ➢ rubella (especially during first trimester) – patent ductus arteriosus, branch pulmonary artery stenosis
➤ maternal drug use
  ➢ alcohol – associated with ventricular septal defects
  ➢ lithium – associated with Ebstein's anomaly
  ➢ cocaine – associated with many congenital heart defects.

CYANOTIC CONGENITAL HEART DISEASE

Cyanotic congenital heart disease is a general term to describe congenital heart defects that result in cyanosis of the newborn. This type of congenital heart defect is less common than acyanotic congenital heart disease.

Central cyanosis is defined as the bluish discolouration of the central mucosal membranes (e.g. tongue) due to an increased concentration of deoxygenated haemoglobin (usually greater than 5 g/dL) in the systemic circulation.

Central cyanosis is associated with low pulse oximeter saturations recordings, and is usually visible at saturations of less than 85%, but this can be difficult to recognise. It is easier to see cyanosis in polycythaemia, and much harder to detect clinically in anaemic children.

Peripheral cyanosis is defined as the bluish discolouration of the peripheries (e.g. hands and feet), which can be due to poor circulating volumes (e.g. hypovolaemia), peripheral vasoconstriction (e.g. in extremes of temperatures), venous congestion (e.g. following delivery of a newborn) or alongside central cyanosis.

Many children will get a peripheral cyanosis around their lips at times of high temperature (e.g. during a viral or bacterial illness). This is not cardiac in nature.

Examples of cyanotic heart defects in descending order of prevalence include:
➤ tetralogy of Fallot
➤ transposition of the great arteries
➤ pulmonary atresia
➤ truncus arteriosus
➤ total anomalous pulmonary venous drainage
➤ tricuspid atresia.

Children become cyanosed with these congenital heart defects for one, or a combination, of two major reasons:
➤ inadequate pulmonary blood flow (e.g. Fallot, pulmonary atresia, tricuspid atresia)
➤ abnormal mixing (e.g. TGA, TAPVD).

Not all neonatal cyanosis is cardiac. Other reasons for neonatal cyanosis include respiratory distress (e.g. meconium aspiration, persistent pulmonary hypertension of the newborn, surfactant deficiency etc.), congenital respiratory defects, sepsis and neurological disease (e.g. seizures).

When faced with 'blue baby' the major decision is whether or not this is likely to be cardiac in cause. Diagnosis can be made using a detailed history, examination and other supplementary investigations available (including a CXR and ECG).

Another useful test is the 'hyperoxia test' (also known as the nitrogen washout test):
➤ obtain an arterial blood gas first
➤ place the neonate in 100% headbox oxygen for 10 to 15 minutes

➤ repeat the arterial blood gas:
  ➤ if the PaO2 has increased greater than 15 to 20 kPa from baseline then it is unlikely to be cardiac in nature
  ➤ if the PaO2 fails to rise, then manage as a cyanotic heart defect (see below).
➤ Note that some people use pulse oximetry to monitor saturations during this test; be aware that this is not a specific test and not recommended.

When a cyanotic heart defect is suspected the management plan is as follows.
➤ Ensure airway and breathing are maintained; this may mean ventilating the child, but not always. A great deal of the time these neonates are blue, but well.
➤ Turn off oxygen if possible; aim for saturations in the mid 70s.
➤ Obtain two vascular access points (and take bloods, including a group and save)
➤ Commence prostaglandin therapy (*see* page 34).
➤ Discuss with paediatric cardiology team for cardiac assessment.

You should assume a neonate with suspected cyanotic heart disease is duct dependent until proven otherwise.

D

Dextrocardia – *see* Isomerism defects
DiGeorge syndrome – *see* Syndromes associated with cardiac
    abnormalities
Double inlet left ventricle (DILV)
Double outlet right ventricle (DORV)
Down syndrome – *see* Syndromes associated with cardiac
    abnormalities
Duct-dependent circulations
Duke's criteria – *see* Infective endocarditis

DOUBLE INLET LEFT VENTRICLE (DILV)

Double inlet left ventricle is a complex defect and falls into the category of single ventricle circulations.

In DILV:

➤ both atrioventricular valves (mitral and tricuspid) open into a common ventricle

➤ there is often a tiny hypoplastic right ventricle with a dominant left ventricle, although sometimes it is difficult to determine if the common ventricle is left or right.

The anatomy of a typical DILV is displayed in Figure 6.18.

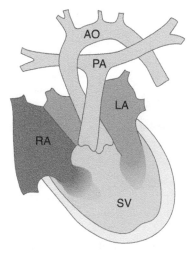

FIGURE 6.18 The anatomy of DILV. SV = systemic ventricle

DILV is different from hypoplastic left/right heart syndromes as in DILV there are two functioning atrioventricular valves.

In hypoplastic hearts there is either mitral atresia/stenosis or tricuspid atresia.

DILV is a cyanotic lesion as all the blood mixes in the common ventricle. As an isolated defect, it is not a duct-dependent circulation.

It is often an antenatal diagnosis, but may present with neonatal cyanosis.

Management is the same as any single ventricle disease.
➤ Initial supportive management as needed.
➤ Staged surgical palliation will create a single ventricle circulation:
  ➤ limiting pulmonary blood flow (e.g. PA band) or augment pulmonary blood flow (Norwood procedure Stage I) depending on the clinical situation
  ➤ Glenn procedure (Stage II) (*see* pages 114 and 147)
  ➤ Fontan procedure (Stage III) (*see* pages 111 and 148).

DOUBLE OUTLET RIGHT VENTRICLE (DORV)

Double outlet right ventricle is a congenital heart disease when both the great arteries (aorta and pulmonary artery) arise from the right ventricle.
➤ More than 50% of the aorta must arise from the RV.

Other congenital heart defects that can be present with DORV include:
➤ ventricular septal defect
➤ pulmonary stenosis (Fallot's type DORV)
➤ the arrangement of the arteries can be normal or transposed (DORV with TGA).

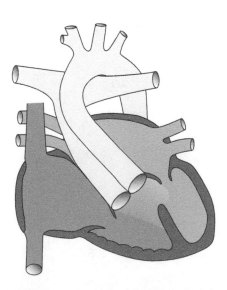

FIGURE 6.19 Double outlet right ventricle (normal arrangement of great vessels, with more than 50% of the aorta arising from the RV)

Incidence is around 12 to 13 cases per 100 000 live births.

DORV can present in a variety of ways:

➤ cyanotic heart defect (especially Fallot's type DORV or DORV with TGA) as there is common mixing of blood and any pulmonary stenosis will shunt blood into the aorta

➤ heart failure due to high pulmonary blood flow (especially normal great arteries with large VSD).

DORV can be associated with:

➤ trisomy 13 (Patau syndrome)

➤ trisomy 18 (Edwards syndrome)

➤ maternal diabetes mellitus

➤ maternal cocaine use.

Management depends on the clinical presentation.

➤ If in heart failure → medical management (*see* page 85) +/– PA band (*see* page 161).

➤ If cyanotic → prostaglandin, consider balloon atrial septostomy +/– BT shunt (*see* page 82).

➤ For all cases surgical repair will be needed. The exact operation will depend greatly on the age of the child, anatomy of the DORV and how they presented.

Clinical features

❯ Antenatal diagnosis

❯ Heart failure (if high pulmonary blood flow)

❯ Cyanosis (if low pulmonary blood flow)

❯ Murmur of VSD

❯ Murmur of pulmonary stenosis (if present)

❯ Features of other syndromes

Investigations

1 CXR may show pulmonary congestion or oligaemia depending on degree of pulmonary blood flow.

2 ECG is often non-specific, but left axis deviation is associated with DORV.

3 Echo is the diagnostic tool.

4 Diagnostic catheterisation may be needed.

DUCT-DEPENDENT CIRCULATIONS

Duct-dependent circulation is a situation in a neonate when the blood flow to either the systemic or pulmonary circulations is dependent upon the patent ductus arteriosus.

Examples of duct-dependent circulations include the following.

➤ Lesions dependent on the PDA to ensure good pulmonary blood flow:

➣ pulmonary atresia

➣ severe forms of tetralogy of Fallot (with severe RV outflow obstruction)

➤ critical pulmonary stenosis
➤ tricuspid atresia.
➤ Lesions dependent on the PDA to ensure good systemic blood flow:
   ➤ coarctation of the aorta
   ➤ critical aortic stenosis
   ➤ hypoplastic left heart syndrome
   ➤ interrupted aortic arch.
➤ Lesions with two parallel circulations:
   ➤ transposition of the great arteries.

Neonates with duct-dependent lesions will appear well initially in the majority of cases. When the duct closes they will present with increasing symptoms until they reach cardiogenic shock when either the systemic circulation or pulmonary circulation is severely compromised.

Management is as follows.
➤ Resuscitation as per neonatal life support (NLS)/APLS guidelines (may need ventilation).
➤ Secure two good vascular access points (e.g. peripheral IV, umbilical venous catheter (UVC), central line).
➤ Commence prostaglandin infusions to assist with duct patency (*see* page 34).
➤ Transfer to a paediatric cardiology unit.
➤ If poor pulmonary blood flow:
   ➤ accept oxygen saturations of 75%
   ➤ may need to alter prostaglandin dose to achieve this
   ➤ may need balloon atrial septostomy to increase mixing (e.g. in TGA)
   ➤ may need urgent BT shunt.
➤ If poor systemic blood flow:
   ➤ may need to hypoventilate and increase CO_2 if high pulmonary blood flow (indicated by high oxygen saturations, cool peripheries, low mean arterial BP)
   ➤ may need urgent corrective procedure (e.g. balloon of aortic valve in critical aortic stenosis or surgical correction of coarctation of aorta).

Clinical features

❯ May have no symptoms in first day or two of life if duct is wide open
❯ Feeding difficulties
❯ Short of breath
❯ Increasing cyanosis
❯ No improvement with oxygen

Investigations

1 Hyperoxia test will demonstrate failure to increase the PaO2 in cyanotic lesions (*see* page 97).
2 Echo will confirm the anatomy of the diagnosis and help assess the size and flow of blood through the PDA.

(*continued*)

Clinical features

> Weak/absent pulse
> Tachycardia
> Respiratory distress
> Poor perfusion
> Murmur may not always be present
> Gallop rhythm (HS I + II + III)
> Hepatomegaly
> Cardiogenic shock
> Clinical features of the cause of the duct-dependent lesion may also be present.

Investigations

3 Other investigations (e.g. ECG, CXR) will be needed and may give an indicator as to the cause of the congenital heart disease.

Ebstein's anomaly
ECG – *see* Chapters 4 and 5, and Appendix
Echo – *see* Chapter 4
Extracorporeal membrane oxygenation (ECMO)
Edwards syndrome – *see* Syndromes associated with cardiac
   abnormalities
Ehlers–Danlos syndrome – *see* Syndromes associated with cardiac
   abnormalities
Eisenmenger syndrome

EBSTEIN'S ANOMALY

Ebstein's anomaly is a rare congenital heart disease affecting the tricuspid valve (Figure 6.20).

➤ Malformation of the tricuspid valve
➤ The valve is rotated and displaced downwards towards the apex of the right ventricle:
   ➤ large right atrium
   ➤ small right ventricle
   ➤ abnormal tricuspid valve with tricuspid regurgitation.

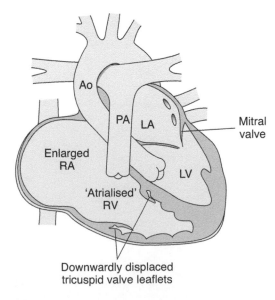

FIGURE 6.20 Morphology of Ebstein's anomaly

The incidence is 3 to 5 per 100 000 live births. There is an association of maternal lithium use during pregnancy and Ebstein's anomaly.

The severity of the Ebstein's anomaly is variable.

➤ Minor forms of Ebstein's have the tricuspid valve only mildly displaced downwards. This may not present until adult life.

➤ Severe forms of Ebstein's have the tricuspid valve inserted down into the base of the right ventricle. This tends to present as a 'blue baby' in the neonatal period.

The clinical features will depend on the severity of tricuspid valve displacement (see below).

The problems with Ebstein's anomaly include:

➤ poor pulmonary blood flow (especially in a neonate) causing cyanosis

➤ the right atria is enlarged and makes the patient prone to arrhythmias

➤ association with Wolff–Parkinson–White syndrome

➤ right ventricular function is often poor (causing RV failure).

Management depends on the severity.

➤ Mild cases can be left with close observation and medical management.

➤ Treatment of any arrhythmias needs to be prompt.

➤ Some centres try to perform surgical repair of the tricuspid valve.

➤ More often these patients need a Glenn shunt to increase pulmonary blood flow or even a full Fontan circulation in severe cases.

Clinical features

A wide spectrum depending on age of presentation and severity

Neonates:

❯ Very unwell

❯ Cyanotic

❯ Poor perfusion

❯ Pansystolic murmur of tricuspid regurgitation

Older children/adults:

❯ Short of breath

❯ Palpitations

❯ Sudden cardiac death

❯ Cyanosis

❯ Clubbing

❯ Wide split first heart sound

❯ Pansystolic murmur of tricuspid regurgitation

Investigations

1 CXR may show cardiomegaly, and in severe cases shows a 'wall to wall' heart.

2 ECG usually shows right atrial hypertrophy (P- pulmonale). It may also show a long PR interval or Wolff–Parkinson–White syndrome or intermittent arrhythmias.

3 Echo shows the displaced tricuspid valve and quantifies the tricuspid regurgitation and RV function.

EXTRACORPOREAL MEMBRANE OXYGENATION (ECMO)

Extracorporeal membrane oxygenation is a longer term form of cardiopulmonary bypass used on PICU to support a child's heart or lungs, or both organs, depending on the clinical situations.

The purpose of ECMO is to rest the lungs and/or heart to allow the child to recover, or receive a definitive form of treatment (e.g. heart transplant).

Only certain centres in the UK offer ECMO as a treatment modality, so transfer to one of these units may be needed in certain cases. ECMO is usually initiated as an emergency or after failure of other conventional treatments.

ECMO has two main types.

➤ Venoarterial (VA)
  ➢ Blood leaves the venous systemic circulation from a cannula placed in the venous system.
  ➢ It passes through an oxygenator where oxygen is added to the blood.
  ➢ It is pumped back into the circulation via a cannula placed in the arterial system to go around the systemic circulation before returning to the venous circulation once again.
  ➢ Both heart and lungs are supported with VA ECMO.
➤ Venovenous (VV)
  ➢ Blood is removed from the venous system, oxygenated and then returned to the venous system to go to the heart.
  ➢ The heart still acts as the pump to move the blood around the body.
  ➢ No cardiac support is offered on VV ECMO, only respiratory support.

A typical ECMO circuit is seen for VA ECMO in Figure 6.21A and VV ECMO in Figure 6.21B.

Indications for ECMO include:

➤ post-cardiac surgery (e.g. failure to come off bypass)
➤ post-cardiac arrest
➤ heart failure
➤ awaiting heart transplantation or Berlin Heart
➤ acute respiratory distress (e.g. bronchiolitis):
  ➢ when oxygenation index is over 40
  ➢ (*Oxygenation Index = [Mean Airway Pressure × FiO$_2$ × 100]/Post-ductal PaO$_2$*)
➤ severe neonatal respiratory distress (with a weight greater than 2 kg):
  ➢ meconium aspiration syndrome
  ➢ persistent pulmonary hypertension of the newborn (PPHN).

EISENMENGER SYNDROME

First described by Eisenmenger in 1897.

A syndrome characterised by the following.

➤ Pulmonary hypertension *secondary* to uncorrected congenital disease.

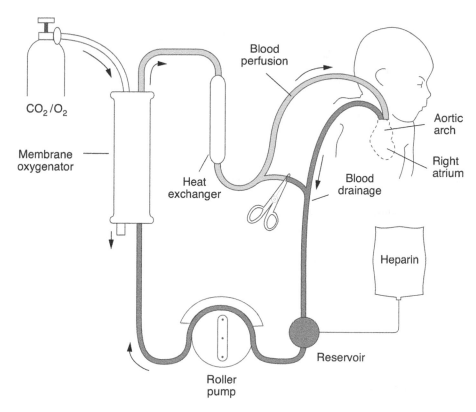

FIGURE 6.21A Venoarterial (VA) ECMO

➤ The congenital heart disease has a left to right shunt for so long that the pulmonary vasculature bed is damaged by the high pulmonary blood flow.
➤ The pulmonary vascular resistance (and pressure) therefore increase, until eventually the pulmonary pressure is supra-systemic.
➤ This causes reversal of the usual left to right cardiac shunt.
➤ The pulmonary vascular damage in this situation is irreversible.

The presence of right to left shunting in uncorrected congenital heart disease and the associated cyanosis is referred to as Eisenmenger syndrome.

Pulmonary arterial pressure (P) is the product of pulmonary blood flow (F) and pulmonary vascular resistance (R):

$$P = R \times F$$

In Eisenmenger syndrome, pulmonary hypertension is as a result of high pulmonary resistance rather than significantly increased pulmonary blood flow.

Pulmonary vascular resistance either remains high or rises through early adult life due to increased shear stress on pulmonary arterioles.

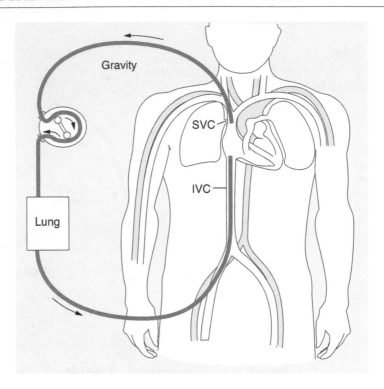

FIGURE 6.21B Venovenous (VV) ECMO

It occurs due to prolonged increased pulmonary pressure resulting in obliterative intimal pulmonary lesions.

It usually presents in early adult life, by which point it is too late to reverse.

Irreversible pulmonary vascular obstruction results in high pulmonary vascular resistance.

It represents an end point at which the pulmonary hypertension is irreversible.

The reason for aggressive treatment of congenital heart disease is to prevent Eisenmenger syndrome.

Cardiac lesions predisposing to Eisenmenger syndrome
➤ ASD
➤ VSD
➤ AVSD
➤ PDA
➤ AV fistula
➤ TAPVD
➤ truncus arteriosus
➤ single ventricle
➤ obstructed pulmonary venous return
➤ mitral stenosis.

Clinical features

> Cyanosis
> Clubbing
> Dyspnoea
> Fatigue
> Cardiac arrhythmia
> Heart failure
> Chest pain
> Syncope
> Haemoptysis
> Right ventricular heave
> Loud, narrowly split second heart sound
> Soft ejection systolic murmur
> Blowing diastolic murmur

Investigations

Investigation	Description
FBC	Polycythaemia
CXR	Enlarged pulmonary vessels
	Prominent right ventricle and right atrium
ECG	Right ventricular hypertrophy
	Tall, spiked P waves
Echo	Thick-walled right ventricle
	Communication between the systemic and pulmonary circulation
Catheter	Bidirectional shunt
	Equal systolic pressures in the systemic and pulmonary circulations
	Decreased arterial oxygen saturation, reflecting the right to left shunt

Management involves prevention with early surgical intervention in infancy. Medical treatment is symptomatic.

For further details on management *see* Pulmonary arterial hypertension on page 159.

Fallot's Tetralogy – *see* Tetralogy of Fallot
Fetal cardiology
Fontan procedure

FETAL CARDIOLOGY

Fetal cardiology is the specialty of diagnosing congenital heart disease in the antenatal period.

In the UK, women have an anomaly scan during pregnancy at 18 to 20 weeks' gestation. This covers all aspects of fetal development, but it is only a screening test.

The anomaly scan for the fetal heart is basic and covers the following.

➤ A four-chamber view (to identify two atria, two ventricles and two atrioventricular valves with a normal offset).

➤ More recently, the ventricular outlet views (to identify a pulmonary artery and aorta that cross over each other with two outlet valves).

While the anomaly scan is useful for detecting many congenital heart lesions, many others are still missed. This is why examination of the newborn is still very important.

Fetal echocardiography is a more detailed assessment of the fetal heart, and is often performed by specialists in fetal cardiology, fetal medicine or paediatric cardiology.

Indications for fetal echocardiography include the following.

➤ Concern with fetal heart rate or rhythm – may indicate fetal SVT or congenital complete heart block.

➤ Abnormal or difficulty with the normal views of the fetal heart on the anomaly scan – may indicate structural heart disease is present in the fetus.

➤ Non-cardiac anomaly found on 18–20 week screening – many non-cardiac anomalies are associated with congenital heart disease.

➤ A family history of congenital heart disease in a first-degree relative – there is an increased risk of congenital heart disease with a positive family history in a first-degree relative, especially if they have required treatment.

➤ A previous fetus with a CHD – there is an increased risk of congenital heart disease.

➤ Maternal diabetes mellitus – maternal diabetes increases the risk of congenital heart disease (especially transposition of the great arteries).

➤ Raised nuchal translucency – associated with congenital heart disease and syndromes (e.g. trisomy 21) that can have associated with congenital heart disease.

➤ Maternal teratogenic drug use – certain drug use is associated with congenital heart disease.

There has been proven benefit to morbidity and mortality in the antenatal diagnosis of congenital heart disease that is suitable for a full biventricular corrective repair (e.g. coarctation of the aorta, transposition of the great arteries).

There is little evidence that the diagnosis of defects needing a univentricular repair (e.g. hypoplastic left heart syndrome) in the antenatal period improves outcome. However, it will allow parents to accept the diagnosis, allow delivery near a cardiac unit and a careful neonatal plan to be implemented in advance.

Fetal arrhythmias can be managed with medication given to the mother (e.g. amiodarone).

Failure to treat fetal arrhythmias can be associated with fetal heart failure and hydrops fetalis.

The fetus with a congenital heart disease has an increased risk of stillbirth or spontaneous miscarriage. Some parents opt for termination of pregnancy in severe heart defects.

Fetal cardiology is an expanding area of medicine.

FONTAN PROCEDURE

The Fontan procedure is a complex operation used in children with severe congenital heart disease which is not suitable for repair into a system with two separate ventricles.

It is also known as total cavopulmonary connection (TCPC).

It is a palliative operation, not a corrective or curative operation.

The Fontan procedure creates a single ventricle circulation (a Fontan circulation) with two separate circulations.

1 The venous return is passive from the body to the pulmonary circulation.
2 The output from the heart is pumped via the single ventricle to the systemic circulation.

The Fontan procedure is usually the third stage of surgery (after a Stage I Norwood and then a Glenn shunt) before the Fontan circulation is complete.

The Fontan procedure involves disconnecting the IVC from the right atria, and connecting it directly to the pulmonary artery. It is important that the pulmonary pressures are low enough to allow the passive venous drainage into the pulmonary artery.

It is usually performed around 3 to 5 years of age. The Glenn shunt by this age is not supplying enough blood from the head and neck to maintain saturations (i.e. the child is outgrowing the Glenn shunt).

After the surgery the child's saturations may be up to 100%, but sometimes a fenestration is left behind as a safety mechanism. (A fenestration is a small communication between the IVC and the RA). If a fenestration is present saturations will be in the low 90%, depending on the size of the fenestration.

The anatomy of a Fontan circulation is shown in Figure 6.22, for a hypoplastic left heart.

However, a similar situation exists in hypoplastic right ventricle (e.g. with tricuspid atresia).

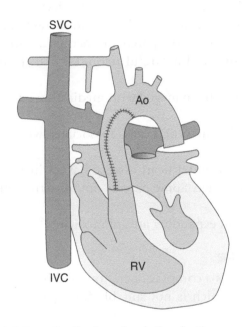

FIGURE 6.22 The anatomy of a Fontan circulation (in the example of a hypoplastic left heart syndrome)

The direction of blood flow around a Fontan circulation is shown in Figure 6.23.

Children with a Fontan circulation or Glenn shunt can deteriorate very rapidly; any symptoms need to be taken seriously. This is discussed under the Norwood procedure and Glenn shunt.

Long-term outlook for people with Fontan circulation is limited:

➤ single ventricle failure
➤ arrhythmia risk high
➤ thromboembolic events.

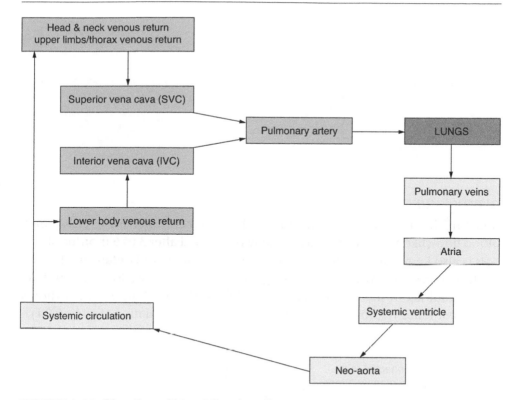

FIGURE 6.23 Direction of blood flow in a Fontan circulation

GLENN SHUNT

A Glenn shunt is another surgical procedure aimed at increasing pulmonary blood flow (like a BT shunt) and is usually performed after 3 to 6 months of age.

It is also known as a bi-directional Glenn shunt or Hemi-Fontan circulation.

The Glenn shunt involves connecting the superior vena cava to the pulmonary artery, resulting in the deoxygenated blood from the head, neck, upper thorax and upper limbs returning directly to the pulmonary circulation (Figure 6.24).

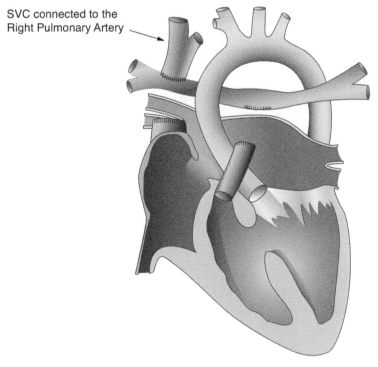

SVC connected to the
Right Pulmonary Artery

FIGURE 6.24 Glenn shunt (in the context of tricuspid atresia)

It is used in situations with low pulmonary blood flow, where it is not possible to correct the heart, and so a single ventricle repair is required. Situations include:

➤ Stage II Norwood for hypoplastic left heart syndrome
➤ hypoplastic right heart syndrome
➤ tricuspid atresia
➤ severe Ebstein's anomaly
➤ double inlet left ventricle
➤ atrioventricular septal defect which is unbalanced (i.e. one ventricle is too small to function suitably when the AVSD is repaired).

The Glenn shunt cannot be performed on a neonate.
➤ The SVC blood flow into the pulmonary artery (PA) is passive and so requires the SVC to be under higher pressure than the PA.
➤ The pulmonary vascular resistance is high in the neonatal period, and so needs to fall.

After the Glenn shunt children will still be cyanosed, as there is not a complete separation of the two circulations yet.
    Potential problems with children with Glenn shunts include:
➤ increased risk of pleural effusions
➤ shunt blockage (e.g. with thrombus – all children on some form of anticoagulation after shunt operations)
➤ increasing desaturations, which can be caused by:
    ➢ child outgrowing the shunt and not enough pulmonary blood flow
    ➢ child being intravascularly volume depleted (e.g. with diarrhoea and vomiting (D&V)) and so not enough circulating volume to drive flow through the shunt, which is based on passive blood flow
    ➢ pulmonary pressures increasing (e.g. with bronchiolitis, pneumonia).

Heart (atrioventricular) blocks
Holt–Oram syndrome – *see* Syndromes associated with cardiac
    abnormalities
Hypertension
Hypoplastic left heart syndrome

HEART (ATRIOVENTRICULAR) BLOCKS

The anatomy and physiology of the electrical conduction system within the heart are discussed in Chapter 2, pages 14 and 23.

A heart block describes a disruption or delay at a point within the electrical conduction system.

Four main heart blocks occur: first degree, second degree, third degree (complete) or bundle branch blocks. Some of these points are discussed in Chapter 4.

First-degree atrioventricular block

A first-degree block is due to a delay in conduction through the atrioventricular node.

It is detected by a prolonged PR interval on the ECG, but every P wave is conducted and followed by a QRS complex (Figure 6.25).

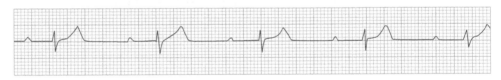

FIGURE 6.25 First-degree AV block (long PR interval, each P wave conducted)

The normal PR interval increases with age. For reference ranges *see* Appendix.

First-degree block does not usually cause any symptoms and does not usually cause bradycardia.

Causes of a first-degree AV block include:
➤ idiopathic (can be normal variant if high vagal tone, such as in athletes)
➤ post-cardiac surgery
➤ atrioventricular septal defects
➤ myocarditis
➤ digoxin toxicity (along with ST depression and inverted/flat T waves)
➤ rheumatic fever
➤ hypokalaemia.

Usually, no treatment is needed other than observation during follow-up, as it does not usually progress to more serious problems.

Second-degree atrioventricular block

Two main types of second-degree AV block exist.
1. Mobitz Type I Block (also known as Wenckebach Block)
   - ➤ The PR interval gradually increases with each beat, until there is non-conduction of a single P wave. After the non-conducted P wave the PR interval resets itself and gradually prolongs with each beat again (Figure 6.26A).

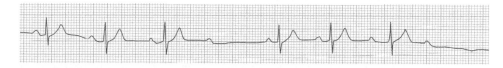

FIGURE 6.26A Second-degree AV Block (Mobitz Type I, Wenckebach block) (Increasing PR interval, with one P wave not conducted)

   - ➤ The block is often quoted as a ratio of non-conducted to conducted beats. For instance, in a 4:3 conduction the fourth P wave is not conducted with three P waves conducted prior to this.
   - ➤ Mobitz Type I is often considered a benign disease, and is seen in normal children when asleep and in athletes (but is less obvious on exercise).
   - ➤ In rare cases it can be pathological, and usually suggests AV node disease and is seen with digoxin toxicity.
   - ➤ If the child is asymptomatic, no intervention other than follow-up is required.
2. Mobitz Type II Block
   - ➤ The PR interval is fixed at a normal value, but there is occasional sudden failure of a P wave to be conducted (Figure 6.26B).
   - ➤ You can often quote the conduction ratio of the number of conducted P waves to the number of non-conducted P waves. For instance a 4:1 block means four P waves are conducted before one P wave is blocked.

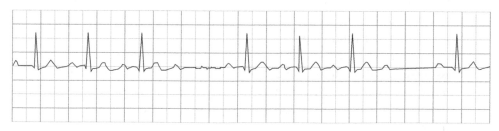

FIGURE 6.26B Second-degree AV Block (Mobitz Type II block) (Fixed PR interval for 3 beats, followed by a single P wave not conducted → 3:1 block)

➤ Although Mobitz Type II block is not common in children, it is usually pathological.
➤ It suggests a conduction delay in the infranodal area (e.g. bundle of His), which means there is risk of progression to third-degree (complete) AV block.
➤ The QRS complex is often wide due to a delay in the conduction bundles.
➤ This type of heart block is an indication for pacemaker insertion.

In a fixed 2:1 block (i.e. two P waves to every QRS) you cannot distinguish between the two types of second-degree AV block, because you do not have multiple PR intervals to assess for prolongation.

Third-degree (complete) atrioventricular block

Third-degree AV block is the complete absence of any electrical conduction from the atria to the ventricles.

As a result of this there is complete electrical dissociation between these chambers. This manifests itself on the ECG as:
➤ regular P-wave activity and regular QRS activity but complete (AV) dissociation between the two waves
➤ regular QRS bradycardia (as the ventricular escape rhythm rate is slow)
➤ a normal or wide QRS, depending on the site of the ventricular escape rhythm.

A typical ECG is demonstrated in Figure 6.27.

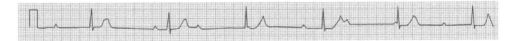

FIGURE 6.27 Third-degree AV block (complete block) (regular P waves at a fast rate, regular QRS complexes at a slow rate but no regularity between the P and QRS deflections)

Third-degree block is always pathological, and often symptomatic with syncope or pre-syncope.

Causes include the following.
➤ Congenital complete heart block:
    ➢ associated with maternal autoantibody disease (e.g. systemic lupus erythematosus, Sjögren's syndrome, rheumatoid arthritis)
    ➢ anti-Ro and anti-La antibodies present in the mother are main risk factors
    ➢ often the bradycardia is well tolerated by the neonate, and intervention is often not required in the neonatal period

> ➤ a pacemaker is usually required as the child grows or in a symptomatic neonate.
- ➤ Post-cardiac surgery:
  - ➤ tetralogy of Fallot
  - ➤ ventricular septal defect
  - ➤ transposition of the great arteries
  - ➤ can occur with any open heart surgery due to damage/oedema of the AV node.
- ➤ Structural heart disease:
  - ➤ isomerism defects
  - ➤ congenitally corrected transposition of the great arteries.
- ➤ Inflammation:
  - ➤ myocarditis
  - ➤ rheumatic fever.
- ➤ Ischaemia/Infarction of conduction system.

Treatment of complete heart block is with a pacemaker (either temporary or permanent). Initial management with an isoprenaline infusion may help while waiting for pacing.

Prognosis is variable. A few children will recover and manage with a temporary pacing system, but many need permanent pacemaker insertion.

Bundle branch blocks

Although not often considered under 'heart blocks', they are a form of conduction delay, but not at the atrioventricular level.

Bundle branch blocks are considered in much more detail in Chapter 4, page 50.

HYPERTENSION

Hypertension in children is defined as a systolic blood pressure of greater than the 95th centile for gender, height and weight of the child.
- ➤ Primary (essential) hypertension → No cause for the raised BP
- ➤ Secondary hypertension → Raised BP is due to an underlying pathology.

Paediatric hypertension tends to be managed by paediatric nephrologists.

It is an increasingly common problem in children and young adults and a cause should always be sought as essential hypertension is rare in infants and young children. It is more common in older children, and is on the increase due to childhood obesity.

BP gradually increases with age. Centile charts and tables exist for children, to help determine if a BP is too high. These are provided in the Appendix.

BP must be recorded carefully using the correct size cuff and manual equipment. If the cuff is too small, there may be an overestimation of BP.

It is important hypertension is taken seriously:
➤ to identify an underlying pathology causing the raised BP
➤ to prevent end organ damage as a consequence of the raised BP.

The heart is an important organ to consider in hypertension:
➤ it can be the cause of the hypertension (e.g. coarctation of the aorta)
➤ it can be damaged by systemic hypertension (e.g. with LV hypertrophy and then failure)
➤ LV hypertrophy is the most common end-organ manifestation in paediatric hypertension.

Causes of secondary hypertension in children and young adults include the following.
➤ Renal:
  ➣ parenchymal disease
  ➣ renal scarring from urinary tract infections
  ➣ glomerular disease
  ➣ renal artery stenosis
  ➣ renal vein thrombosis
  ➣ Wilms' tumour.
➤ Cardiac:
  ➣ coarctation of the aorta (typically post-ductal) – *see* page 93.
➤ Endocrine:
  ➣ Cushing's disease
  ➣ primary hyperaldosteronism
  ➣ phaeochromocytoma.
➤ Neurological:
  ➣ raised intracranial pressure (e.g. brain tumour).
➤ Pharmacological:
  ➣ steroid use
  ➣ illicit drug use.
➤ Miscellaneous:
  ➣ pain
  ➣ anxiety
  ➣ incorrect recordings!

Studies have demonstrated renal parenchymal abnormalities are the commonest cause of secondary hypertension overall in children.
When taking a history and examining a child with hypertension, you must guide the encounter to help differentiate the causes from the above list.
Management is very dependent on the cause.
➤ Treat underlying cause.
➤ Close assessment for evidence of end organ damage.

➤ Treat any end organ damage if possible.
➤ Antihypertensive medications.

End organ damage of hypertension is as follows.
1 Renal → Renal impairment/failure, proteinuria.
2 Cardiac → LV hypertrophy, heart failure, vascular damage, ischaemic heart disease.
3 Neurological → Stroke, transient ischaemic attacks, intracranial bleeds.
4 Eyes → Retinal haemorrhage and exudates.
5 Respiratory → Pulmonary hypertension.

Hypertensive emergency

A hypertensive emergency is when the BP is elevated (usually above the 99th centile) with evidence of end organ damage.
   Rare in paediatrics, but very important.
   Management:
➤ seek specialist help
➤ treat the cause
➤ deal with the end organ dysfunction
➤ decrease BP:
   ➤ need to drop slowly – do not decrease more than 10% initially
   ➤ use short-acting antihypertensive medications (IV labetolol or hydralazine)
➤ may need to involve PICU – risk of seizures.

Clinical features

❯ Asymptomatic
❯ Symptoms and signs of the underlying cause
❯ Headaches
❯ Lethargy
❯ Blurred vision
❯ Epistaxis
❯ Hypertension
❯ Obesity/Raised BMI
❯ *Acanthosis nigricans*
❯ Evidence of end organ damage

Investigations

1 Regular BP recordings (may use an ambulatory BP monitor).
2 Investigate as indicated for the cause. This may need a multidisciplinary approach (e.g. endocrine investigations, renal investigations).
3 An echo is important to look for coarctation of the aorta and evidence of end organ damage to the heart.
4 Asses for evidence of end organ damage:
   a. ECG (for LVH)
   b. CXR (for cardiomegaly)
   c. Echo (for LVH)
   d. Fundoscopy (for retinal damage)
   e. Renal investigations: (i.) U&E (ii.) Urinalysis.

HYPOPLASTIC LEFT HEART SYNDROME (HLHS)

Hypoplastic left heart syndrome (Figure 6.28) is a severe congenital heart disease consisting of the spectrum of:

1 Mitral atresia (or severe mitral stenosis)
2 Tiny, insignificant hypoplastic left ventricle
3 Aortic atresia (or severe aortic stenosis)
4 Hypoplasia of the ascending aorta.

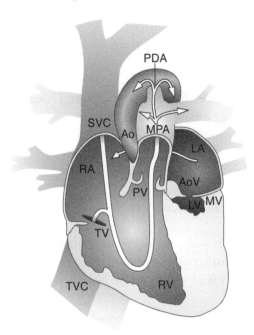

FIGURE 6.28 The anatomy of hypoplastic left heart syndrome

It is a rare disorder (266 cases per 1 million live births), but is a significant part of paediatric cardiology workload as these children can be very ill and need multiple interventions.

Many cases of HLHS are diagnosed antenatally on obstetric anomaly scans. Only a few cases are diagnosed in the postnatal period. As a result, many families choose to terminate before delivery.

This circulation is an example of duct-dependent systemic circulation (*see* page 101).

Initial management is with prostaglandin therapy (*see* page 34), with careful monitoring and support of respiratory and circulatory function. These babies are usually well in the first 24 hours of life.

Long-term management is with the surgical Norwood procedure (*see* page 146), but this is only palliative. Some of these children die during the surgery. Those that make it to adulthood die young or need a heart transplant.

Clinical features

> Antenatal diagnosis (asymptomatic)
> If unwell:
  ✓ Tachypnoea
  ✓ Cyanosis
  ✓ Weak/absent peripheral pulses
  ✓ Poor perfusion
  ✓ Tachycardia
  ✓ Hepatomegaly

Investigations

1 ECG can show a sinus tachycardia with dominant RV forces, and reduced LV forces.
2 CXR can be normal or show cardiomegaly with heart failure.
3 Echo will be diagnostic.

Infective endocarditis (IE)
Innocent murmurs
Interrupted aortic arch (IAA)
Isomerism defects and dextrocardia

INFECTIVE ENDOCARDITIS (IE)

Infective endocarditis is defined as an infection of the endocardial surface of the heart.

In children it most commonly occurs as a complication of congenital heart disease or prosthetic valves, but it can occur in children with structurally normal hearts.

There is an increased risk with intravascular devices, intravenous drug use and cardiac lesions with a high-velocity blood flow such as ventricular septal defects.

Pathophysiology

All cases of infective endocarditis develop from a commonly shared process, as follows.

1   Bacteraemia that delivers the organisms to the surface of the valve.
2   Adherence of the organisms.
3   Eventual invasion of the valvular leaflets.

A high-velocity flow through a stenotic or incompetent valve causes turbulence.

This turbulence damages the endothelium, to which platelets and fibrin adhere → thrombotic endocardial lesions.

Circulating bacteria and inflammatory cells adhere to and grow in these thrombi, forming infected vegetation.

Once vegetation forms, the constant blood flow may result in embolisation to virtually any organ in the body.

An immunological response is produced.

Epidemiology

US figures: 1 case per 1000 paediatric hospital admissions.

Incidence remained unchanged over last 40 years.

No racial/gender predilection is observed.

IE is most frequently observed in adults, but the incidence in children with CHD or central indwelling venous catheters continues to rise.

The classic clinical presentation and clinical course of IE has been characterised as either acute or subacute:

Acute	Sub-acute
Toxic	Non-specific flu-like illness
Febrile – high grade	Symptoms present for greater than 2 weeks
Rigors	More common in patients with an underlying congenital heart disease
Rapid onset of congestive heart failure	Not usually associated with rigors
Symptoms present for less than 2 weeks	
IV drug abuse may be elicited	
Staphylococcus aureus most commonly found organism	

Organisms

➤ *Staphylococcus aureus*
➤ A, C, G streptococci
➤ *Streptococcus viridans/S. oralis*
➤ *Haemophilus, Actinobacillus* – neonates, immunocompromised children. *Enterococci* is a rare but dangerous causative organism.

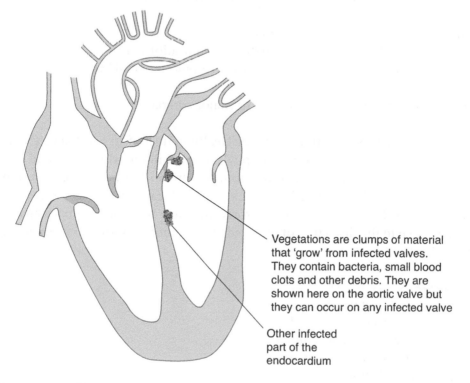

Vegetations are clumps of material that 'grow' from infected valves. They contain bacteria, small blood clots and other debris. They are shown here on the aortic valve but they can occur on any infected valve

Other infected part of the endocardium

FIGURE 6.29 Heart with infective endocarditis

Duke's criteria:
Clinical criteria for definite infective endocarditis:
➤ one major or,
➤ one major and three minor or,
➤ five minor criteria.

Major:
➤ Positive blood culture (2 separate cultures taken at different times and sites for an organism typically associated with endocarditis)
➤ Positive echo findings (mass adherent to the endocardium, abscess formation or increasing new valvular regurgitation).

Minor:
➤ Predisposition to endocarditis (e.g. congenital heart disease)
➤ fever: greater than 38 degrees
➤ vascular phenomena: Janeway lesions
➤ immunologic phenomena – Osler's nodes, Roth spots
➤ positive blood culture findings without meeting the major criteria above.

Management
Broad spectrum IV antibiotics at high bactericidal levels usually for duration of 4–6 weeks.
Surgical intervention may be necessary.
Prognosis largely depends upon whether complications arise.
Prevention involves antibiotic prophylaxis, scrupulous dental hygiene and patient education.
Positive blood culture not satisfying the major criteria

Prophylaxis: The National Institute for Health and Clinical Excellence (NICE) no longer recommends antibiotic prophylaxis for children with congenital heart disease. However, recommendations from the British Cardiac Society Working Group state that: 'Those at risk of developing endocarditis should receive antibiotic therapy before undergoing a procedure likely to result in a bacteraemia.' This is down to the discretion of the paediatric cardiologist for major congenital heart disease.

High risk: Class I:
➤ prosthetic heart valves
➤ previous infective endocarditis
➤ complex cyanotic congenital heart disease
➤ transposition of the great arteries
➤ tetralogy of Fallot
➤ surgically constructed systemic pulmonary shunts or conduits

➤ mitral valve prolapse with clinically significant mitral regurgitation or thickened valve leaflets.

Clinical features

> Fever 85%–99%
> Fatigue/malaise
> Chills
> Sweats
> Anorexia
> Cough
> Headache
> Myalgia
> Arthralgia
> Classic skin lesions – Osler's nodes, Janeway lesions, splinter haemorrhages

Investigations

> FBC
> CRP, ESR
> Blood culture from three different sites at different times
> Echocardiogram
> ECG
> CXR
> Urine – microscopic haematuria

INNOCENT MURMURS

Innocent murmurs in children are very common and frequently encountered by all paediatricians and general practitioners. They are reported to occur in up to 40% of children.

The murmur occurs due to audible flow of blood within the heart for many reasons (thin chest wall; anaemia; pyrexia; intercurrent infection).

Despite the fact that these children have a structurally normal heart, great anxiety exists within the family without a clear explanation of the 'normality' of these murmurs in children.

Innocent murmurs have specific clinical features (see below). However, innocent murmurs are *never*:

➤ found only in the diastolic period
➤ associated with a thrill
➤ associated with abnormal heart sounds or other cardiac abnormality on examination
➤ found in a symptomatic child until cardiac pathology is excluded
➤ associated with abnormal investigations until cardiac pathology is excluded.

Because innocent murmurs are all due to flow, they will characteristically vary with the alteration of the child's posture (e.g. from lying down to standing up).

Innocent murmurs have been described into different types. In reality it does not matter which type of innocent murmur it is, but people will often talk about the following classification.

1 Still's murmur:
   ➤ low-pitched, vibratory or 'squeaky' type murmur
   ➤ loudest at mid to lower left sternal border
   ➤ more common aged 3 to adolescence.

2   Pulmonary flow murmurs:
  ➤ high-pitched, harsher murmur
  ➤ loudest at upper left sternal border
  ➤ more common in pre-term infants (with physiological pulmonary artery branch stenosis), adolescence or when cardiac output increases with higher flow through the pulmonary valve (e.g. anaemia, pyrexia).

3   Venous hum:
  ➤ low-pitched, continuous murmur
  ➤ due to venous return from the vena cava (especially SVC) to the right atria
  ➤ loudest at the upper right sternal edge, under the clavicle
  ➤ classically disappears when the neck veins are gently compressed or when getting the child to look down and to the side.

Management is plenty of reassurance to the family and no follow-up is needed. It is important to mention to them that when their child develops a temperature the murmur will get louder (as flow will increase).

Clinical features

> Asymptomatic child
> Murmur
  ✓ Soft and less than 2–3/6 systolic (never have an associated thrill)
  ✓ Varies with posture
  ✓ Always systolic, or continuous in venous hum (never isolated diastolic)
  ✓ Often localised (especially left sternal edge)
  ✓ Associated with normal heart sounds

Remainder of the cardiovascular examination is normal (e.g. good volume pulses)

Investigations

1   ECG is normal.
2   CXR is normal.
3   Echo is normal.

No further investigations are required in innocent murmur assessment.

INTERRUPTED AORTIC ARCH (IAA)

Interrupted aortic arch is a congenital defect where there is no continuity between two segments of the aortic arch.

The distal end of the aorta is connected to the main pulmonary artery by a patent ductus arteriosus.

A classification system exists based on where the interruption within the arch

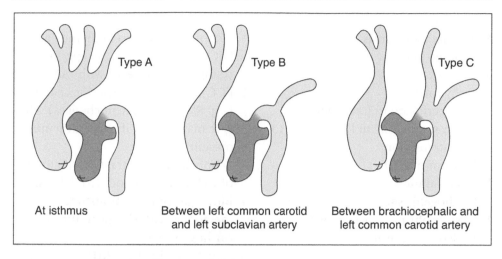

FIGURE 6.30 The classification of IAA

occurs relative to the head and neck branches on the aortic arch (types A–C; type B is the most common type). This is demonstrated in Figure 6.30.

IAA is a neonatal duct-dependent lesion with high mortality without treatment. Median age of death is 10 days old without treatment.

IAA accounts for 1.3% of congenital heart defects (approximately 2 cases per 100 000 births).

It can be associated with syndromes including:

➤ DiGeorge (22q11 microdeletion) – up to 50% of children with IAA have this syndrome
➤ velocardiofacial syndrome
➤ CHARGE syndrome.

IAA is often associated with other structural heart lesions:

➤ ventricular septal defects (in 90% of IAA cases)
➤ truncus arteriosus
➤ transposition of the great arteries.

Neonates often present with cardiogenic shock (similar to coarctation of the aorta) when the PDA closes (see below).

Management of IAA is as follows.

➤ Resuscitation and stabilisation in accordance to APLS/NLS guidelines.
➤ Commence IV prostaglandin (*see* page 34).
➤ Arrange transfer to paediatric cardiology centre.
➤ Surgical correction of the aortic arch is definitive treatment.

Clinical features

> Antenatal diagnosis
> Poor feeding
> Lethargy
> Tachycardia
> Poor perfusion in lower body
> Lower saturations in limbs distal to the interruption
> Murmur of VSD
> Heart failure
> Cardiogenic shock
> Dysmorphism associated with DiGeorge syndrome

Investigations

1 CXR may show absent thymus with DiGeorge syndrome. No specific changes on CXR exist with IAA.
2 ECG often has non-specific changes (e.g. RVH, ST segment changes). The QTc may be long if hypocalcaemia present.
3 Echo will demonstrate the anatomy of IAA and any associated defects.
4 Blood gas often demonstrates metabolic acidosis due to the cardiogenic shock.
5 Genetic testing for 22q11 microdeletion.
6 Calcium levels should be checked (hypocalcaemia associated with DiGeorge syndrome).

ISOMERISM DEFECTS AND DEXTROCARDIA

In cardiac anatomy, it is important to consider where the heart is within the chest and identify the left and right side, before going on to determine the internal cardiac anatomy.

This is a short summary of these complex defects.

Dextrocardia and dextroposition

Dextroposition means that the heart is moved towards the right side of the chest, but the apex of the heart is still pointing to the left.

True dextrocardia means that the apex of the heart is pointing to the right side of the chest.

Dextrocardia is a very non-specific word, and you should be clear of its definition when using this term. For instance, a tension pneumothorax on the left side may push the mediastinum and heart to the right, but the apex is still pointing to the left. This is not dextrocardia; it is dextroposition.

Dextrocardia can be:

➤ isolated (i.e. only the heart is in abnormal position)
➤ Associated with situs inversus (i.e. all the other organs are in the mirror image position).

A normal heart can be abnormally located, although if the heart is abnormally located, close attention must be paid to the rest of the cardiac anatomy.

➤ Isolated dextrocardia is more likely to be associated with significant congenital heart disease than dextrocardia with situs inversus.

Kartagener's syndrome (also known as primary ciliary dyskinesia) is the triad association of:
➤ dextrocardia with situs inversus
➤ bronchiectasis
➤ chronic sinusitis
➤ plus other associated features secondary to ciliary dyskinesia.

A CXR will demonstrate the orientation of the heart in the chest.
   ECG will also help identify dextrocardia:
➤ inverted P waves in lead I
➤ absent R wave progression in chest leads.

Isomerism defects

Isomerism means 'mirror image'.
   Defects associated with isomerism are usually very complex.
   Right atrial isomerism means that there are two right atria and no left atria:
➤ i.e. mirror image right atria
➤ also known as asplenia syndrome because the spleen is usually absent
➤ associated with anomalous pulmonary venous drainage (as no left atria to drain into)
➤ often has two SA nodes.

Left atrial isomerism means that there are two left atria and no right atria:
➤ i.e. mirror image left atria
➤ also known as polysplenia syndrome because multiple, small less effective spleens are present
➤ often no SA node and can have associated conduction defects.

Jervell and Lange–Nielsen syndrome – *see* Syndromes associated with cardiac abnormalities

Jatene procedure – *see* Arterial switch procedure

Jones criteria – *see* Rheumatic fever

KAWASAKI DISEASE

First described by Tomisaku Kawasaki in 1967 who described distinctive changes in 50 children from Tokyo.

Also known as acute febrile mucocutaneous syndrome; it is an acute febrile vasculitic syndrome of early childhood.

It is the second commonest vasculitic illness in childhood.

A vasculitis affecting small and medium-sized arteries.

Mainly affects children from 6 months to 4 years old.

Affected children usually present with prolonged high-grade fever, rash and conjunctival injection.

A third of children develop coronary artery aneurysms within the first 6 weeks of illness.

With prompt treatment the prognosis is good, with UK mortality figures estimated at around 2%.

Diagnosis

Clinical diagnostic criteria: There is no one specific diagnostic test for Kawasaki disease and therefore children must meet the clinical diagnostic criteria.

Criterion	Description
Fever	Of 5 days' duration plus four of the following:
Conjunctivitis	conjunctival infection or injection
Cervical lymphadenopathy	greater than 1.5 cm
Rash	polymorphous
Mucous membrane changes	strawberry red tongue, dry, red, cracked lips, pharyngeal injection
Changes to extremities	erythema and oedema of hands and feet, peeling of fingertip skin

Incomplete cases: These children have a prolonged fever and clinically appear to have Kawasaki disease, although they do not fit the diagnostic criteria. They have no other identified cause for their illness.

Differential diagnoses include:
➤ staphylococcal scalded skin syndrome

➤ scarlet fever
➤ toxic shock syndrome.

Investigations

Blood investigations reveal a neutrophilia, raised CRP and ESR. Thrombocytosis is found, but not usually until the second week of illness.

Cerebrospinal fluid (CSF) analysis may show predominantly lymphocytes as seen in children with an aseptic meningitis.

Cardiac complications:

➤ coronary artery aneurysms
➤ myocarditis
➤ cardiac failure
➤ pericarditis.

Other systemic complications:

➤ aseptic meningitis
➤ sterile pyuria
➤ septic arthritis
➤ hepatitis (with deranged LFTs)
➤ uveitis
➤ gastroenteritis
➤ hydrops of the gallbladder.

Management

Aspirin given at high dose for 2 weeks followed by a further 6 months at a reduced dose.

High anti-inflammatory doses are given to reduce the risk of thrombosis.

Intravenous gamma globulin (IVIG) is given as a single high-dose infusion which aims to reduce the incidence of coronary artery aneurysms if given within the first 10 days of illness.

All affected children need an echocardiogram and an ECG. These should be repeated at regular intervals as part of follow-up.

Clinical features	Investigations
❯ Fever	❯ FBC
❯ Conjunctivitis	❯ CRP, ESR, *anti-neutrophil cytoplasmic antibodies* (ANCA)
❯ Strawberry red tongue	
❯ Polymorphous rash	❯ LFT
❯ Peeling of fingers and toes	❯ ECG, Echo
❯ Mucous membrane changes	❯ Blood culture
❯ Cracked red lips	❯ Urine microscopy
❯ Cervical lymphadenopathy	❯ +/− lumbar puncture (LP) as part of full septic screen
❯ Oedematous hands and feet	

Leopard syndrome – *see* Syndromes associated with cardiac
   abnormalities
Long QT syndrome – *see under* QT

Marfan syndrome – *see* Syndromes associated with cardiac
   abnormalities
Mitral regurgitation (MR)
Mitral stenosis (MS)
Murmurs
Mustard procedure
Myocarditis

MITRAL REGURGITATION (MR)

Mitral regurgitation is the term used to describe a leak of blood in the opposite direction to normal across the mitral valve (i.e. from the left ventricle to the left atria) (Figure 6.31).

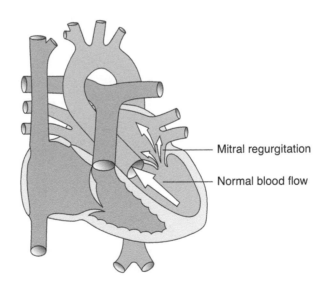

FIGURE 6.31 Mitral regurgitation

When MR is present in children, a cause should be carefully investigated (Figure 6.32). Often in children, MR is a sign of another pathology.

Causes of MR can be classified based on the anatomical location of the disease/damage:

➤ diseases or damage of the mitral valve leaflets
➤ diseases or damage of the mitral valve annulus
➤ diseases or damage of the chordae tendinae or papillary muscles.

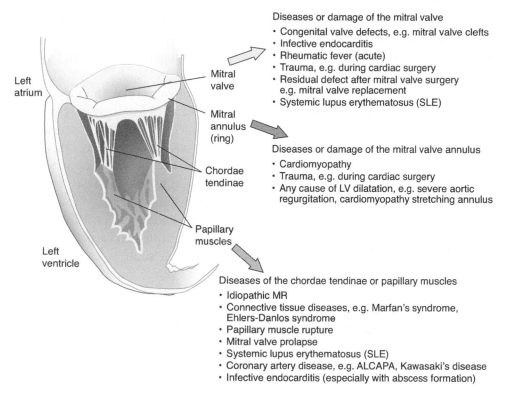

Diseases or damage of the mitral valve
• Congenital valve defects, e.g. mitral valve clefts
• Infective endocarditis
• Rheumatic fever (acute)
• Trauma, e.g. during cardiac surgery
• Residual defect after mitral valve surgery
  e.g. mitral valve replacement
• Systemic lupus erythematosus (SLE)

Diseases or damage of the mitral valve annulus
• Cardiomyopathy
• Trauma, e.g. during cardiac surgery
• Any cause of LV dilatation, e.g. severe aortic
  regurgitation, cardiomyopathy stretching annulus

Diseases of the chordae tendinae or papillary muscles
• Idiopathic MR
• Connective tissue diseases, e.g. Marfan's syndrome,
  Ehlers-Danlos syndrome
• Papillary muscle rupture
• Mitral valve prolapse
• Systemic lupus erythematosus (SLE)
• Coronary artery disease, e.g. ALCAPA, Kawasaki's disease
• Infective endocarditis (especially with abscess formation)

Left atrium

Left ventricle

Mitral valve

Mitral annulus (ring)

Chordae tendinae

Papillary muscles

FIGURE 6.32 The anatomy of the mitral valve apparatus and the causes of MR

The symptoms of MR will vary depending on the age of the child, the underlying cause of the MR, the severity of the MR and the speed of onset of the MR:
➤ acute onset MR is poorly tolerated and these children often have pulmonary hypertension and heart failure
➤ chronic MR is usually well tolerated and often has minimal symptoms.

Severe MR will result in a dilated left atria. This predisposes to atrial fibrillation, although it is rare in children.

The management of MR includes the following.
➤ Careful investigation to identify a cause of the MR.
➤ Careful follow-up and monitoring in mild cases.
➤ Treating any underlying causes (e.g. mitral valve clefts, cardiomyopathy etc.).
➤ Treating any associated complications (e.g. AF, heart failure, thromboembolic risk).
➤ In some cases a mitral valve replacement is needed.

Clinical features

> Asymptomatic
> Mild shortness of breath
> Reduced exercise tolerance
> Lethargy
> Palpitations
> Heart failure (acute or chronic)
> Murmur of MR
  ✓ Pansystolic murmur
  ✓ Loudest at the apex
  ✓ Radiates to axilla

Features of an underlying cause (e.g. Marfan syndrome)

Investigations

1 ECG is often normal. In more severe cases of MR there may be left atrial enlargement (p-mitrale). AF may be seen.
2 CXR is often normal. In more severe cases of MR there may be cardiomegaly. Pulmonary oedema can be seen in acute onset cases.
3 Echo can identify the presence of MR and its severity. The haemodynamic effect of the MR can be seen, and possible causes identified. 3D echo can be especially helpful.

MITRAL STENOSIS (MS)

Mitral stenosis is the narrowing of the left atrioventricular (mitral) valve.
    It is not a common defect; regurgitation at the mitral valve level is much more common
    Mitral stenosis results in an obstruction of flow from the left atrium to the left ventricle.
    Causes of mitral stenosis include the following.
➤ Acquired as a complication of rheumatic fever (*see* page 173) (commonest cause, usually seen at least 20 years following the initial disease).
➤ Congenital isolated mitral valve stenosis.
➤ Associated with other congenital heart defects:
  ➢ hypoplastic left heart syndrome variants
  ➢ Shone's Complex: coarctation of the aorta; subaortic membrane (causing LV outflow tract obstruction); parachute mitral valve (a defect of the mitral valve); supravalvular mitral ring/stenosis (causing LV inflow obstruction).
➤ Associated with some metabolic diseases.

Complications of mitral stenosis include:
➤ raised left atrial pressures
➤ risk of atrial fibrillation (and so thromboembolic events)
➤ risk of pulmonary venous hypertension
➤ reduced cardiac output.

Treatment depends on the severity of the stenosis.
➤ Mild cases may only need observation.
➤ May consider balloon dilatation of the MV.

➤ Mitral valve replacement.
➤ Treat any associated complications (e.g. AF, heart failure).

Clinical features

> Asymptomatic
> Features of heart failure or pulmonary hypertension
> Shortness of breath (worse with tachycardia)
> Palpitations
> Haemoptysis
> Raised jugular venous pressure (JVP)
> Displaced, tapping apex beat
> Loud first heart sound (+/– opening snap)
> Murmur
  ✓ Mid-diastolic rumble
  ✓ Low-pitched
  ✓ Best heard over apex
  ✓ Need patient in left lateral position
  ✓ Use the bell of the stethoscope
> Irregularly irregular pulse (sometimes)
> Adults display mitral facies (flushed cheeks, due to chronic mitral stenosis leading to vasoconstriction and low cardiac output)

Investigations

1 CXR is can be normal. It may show left atrial enlargement (identified by a second shadow within the heart shadow). Features of pulmonary venous congestion may be present.
2 ECG can be normal, but may show left atrial hypertrophy (P-mitrale). AF may be seen in some cases.
3 Echo will demonstrate the mitral stenosis and its severity. It will identify other congenital heart defects.
4 Diagnostic cardiac catheterisation may be used to assess the severity of the stenosis.

MURMURS

A murmur results from turbulent blood flow and has the greatest intensity at the site of disturbed flow.

Murmurs should be described as to their:

➤ intensity
➤ quality
➤ pitch
➤ radiation
➤ site
➤ timing (Figures 6.33 and 6.34).

The intensity (loudness) of a systolic murmur can be described using the conventional grading scale of 1–6. (Note that diastolic murmurs are graded 1 to 4).

Grade	Description
1	Very quiet
2	Soft
3	Audible all over the praecordium. *No thrill*
4	Loud with a palpable thrill
5	Very loud, with a thrill
6	Very loud, with thrill, may be audible to naked ear

Depending on the timing of the murmur in relation to the first and second heart sounds, systolic murmurs can be classified into:
➤ ejection systolic
➤ pansystolic.

A continuous murmur is a systolic murmur that continues into diastole. This indicates continuous flow as in a PDA or a venous hum.

In congenital heart disease most murmurs are systolic in timing, and it is rare to have a diastolic murmur without an associated systolic murmur.

An isolated diastolic murmur is always pathological.

Diastolic murmurs are usually classified as early, mid or late diastolic.

The innocent murmur

They are commonly heard in children and adolescents and originate from the normal turbulence during ejection into the pulmonary artery.

Characteristics:
➤ high-pitched
➤ early systolic
➤ grades 1–3
➤ soft
➤ change in intensity with altered position.

For further details *see* page 127 under Innocent murmurs.

Venous hum

A venous hum is produced by turbulence of blood in the jugular venous system. It is a common insignificant bruit heard during childhood. The soft humming is heard during systole and diastole and the intensity varies with altered position.

For further details *see* page 127 under Innocent murmurs.

Diagrams showing timing murmurs in relation to heart sounds

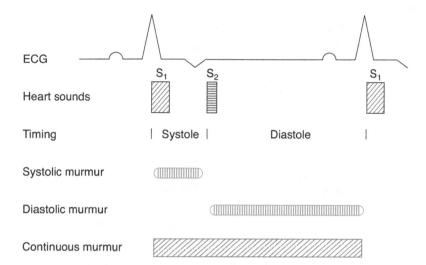

FIGURE 6.33

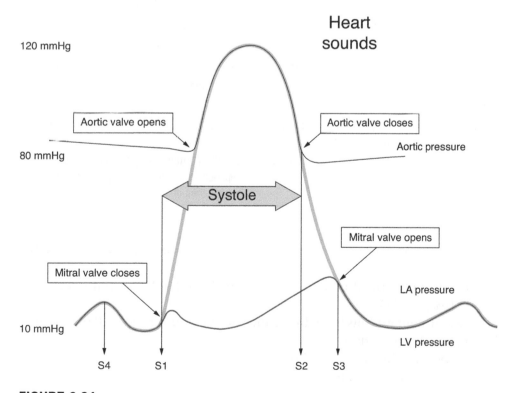

FIGURE 6.34

Cardiac lesion	Heart sounds	Murmur
Acyanotic		
ASD	Wide and fixed second heart sounds	Ejection systolic murmur Upper left sternal edge (LSE)
VSD	Loud second heart sounds (pulmonary artery hypertension)	Pansystolic Lower LSE +/- apical mid-diastolic murmur if large shunt
AVSD	Fixed second heart sounds or loud second heart sound depending on the size of the atrial and ventricular components of the defect	Systolic murmur Lower LSE Radiates to the axilla Mid-diastolic flow murmur Lower LSE
PDA	Loud second heart sound	Continuous systolic murmur Upper LSE
Pulmonary stenosis	An ejection click soon after first heart sound	Ejection systolic murmur Upper LSE radiates to back
Aortic stenosis	Ejection click (mobile valve leaflet)	Ejection systolic murmur Upper right sternal edge (RSE) Radiates to the neck
Coarctation of the aorta	Ejection click if bicuspid aortic valve	Mid-systolic Loud at the back
Cyanotic		
TGA	Single accentuated second heart sound	May have murmur of VSD or associated defect
Tetralogy of Fallot	Single second heart sound	Systolic murmur – length and intensity depends on the degree of right ventricular outflow tract obstruction

MUSTARD PROCEDURE

The Mustard procedure used to be the surgical treatment for transposition of the great arteries.

It is rarely performed now, having been replaced by the arterial switch procedure (*see* page 71).

However, young adults born during the late 1980s and 1990s still survive after having had this procedure.

The operation involves the following.

➤ Inserting a intra-atrial baffle.

➤ This baffle directs the vena caval blood to the left atrium:
  ➤ this then enters into the left ventricle
  ➤ it exits the LV via the pulmonary artery to the lungs.

➤ The baffle directs the oxygenated pulmonary venous blood to the right
   atrium:
   ➤ this then enters into the right ventricle
   ➤ it exits the RV via the aorta to the systemic circulation.
➤ Therefore it attempts to correct the transposition at an atrial level.

The anatomy is demonstrated in Figure 6.35.

Patients with the Mustard procedure are prone to arrhythmias due to disruption of the atrial conduction system by the surgery, sudden cardiac death and
ventricular failure, as the systemic ventricle is actually the right ventricle and cannot deal with systemic pressures indefinitely.

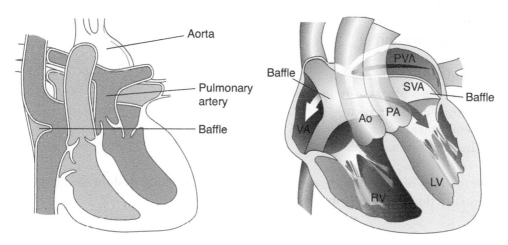

FIGURE 6.35 The Mustard procedure   **FIGURE 6.36** The Senning procedure

Senning procedure

This is another procedure for TGA, similar to the Mustard procedure. It was super-
seded by the Mustard procedure, and is rarely performed.

It is another way of attempting to correct for the transposition at the atrial level.

The differences between the Mustard and Senning procedures relate to
technicalities and are not relevant for this book. The anatomy is very similar
(Figure 6.36).

Long-term complications are the same as for the Mustard procedure.

MYOCARDITIS

Myocarditis involves inflammation of the myocardium. An inflammatory infil-
trate of the myocardium with necrosis and/or degeneration of adjacent myocytes.

Usually, it is a direct result of a viral infection of the myocardium.

In a child it is usually preceded by an upper respiratory tract infection and fever.

They present with a short history of fever, shortness of breath and signs of heart failure.

The ECG shows decreased voltage, prolonged QT interval with flattening of the T waves.

The chest X-ray shows cardiomegaly with pulmonary venous congestion.

Echocardiogram shows poor ventricular contractility, particularly on the left side, with dilated cardiac chambers.

Those with advanced cardiomyopathy, left bundle branch block and low ejection fraction have increased risk of needing heart transplantation.

All these patients require care within a tertiary level cardiac unit. Specific treatment will depend on the clinical and investigative findings, although it may consist of:

➤ inotropic support
➤ cardiac monitoring
➤ diuretics
➤ fluid restriction
➤ avoiding β-blockers in the acute phase of illness
➤ supplemental oxygen
➤ temporary pacing
➤ heart transplant assessment.

The majority of patients recover without any residual cardiac dysfunction; approximately a third will develop dilated cardiomyopathy.

Causes

Viral:	Epstein-Barr	**Other:**	Thyrotoxicosis
	Coxsackie		IBD – ulcerative colitis, Crohn's disease, SLE
	Mumps		
	CMV		Kawasaki disease
	RSV		Sarcoidosis
Bacterial:	Staphylococcal	**Fungal:**	Candida
	Streptococcal		Aspergillosis
	Mycoplasma		Histoplasmosis
	Tuberculosis		
Drugs:	Penicillin Sulfonamides Chloramphenicol Phenytoin Carbamazepine		

Cardiac complications:

➤ arrhythmias
➤ left bundle branch block
➤ congestive heart failure
➤ cardiogenic shock
➤ advanced dilated cardiomyopathy.

Lieberman classification

Type of myocarditis	Features
Fulminant	Preceded by viral illness. Rapid onset of severe cardiovascular compromise with ventricular dysfunction. May result in death.
Acute	Gradual onset of illness with established ventricular dysfunction. May progress to dilated cardiomyopathy.
Chronic active	Gradual onset with relapsing and remitting course. Associated with chronic inflammatory changes.
Chronic persistent	Persistent symptoms: chest pain, palpitations without ventricular dysfunction.

Clinical features

> Dyspnoea
> Tachycardia
> Fever
> Soft heart sounds
> Gallop rhythm
> New cardiac murmurs

Investigations

> FBC
> U&Es
> CRP, ESR, ASOT
> Blood culture
> CXR
> ECG, ECHO
> Cardiac enzymes – troponin I and T
> Creatine kinase levels
> Serum viral antibody titres
> +/– endomyocardial biopsy

Noonan syndrome – *see* Syndromes associated with cardiac
    abnormalities
Norwood staged procedure for hypoplastic left heart

NORWOOD STAGED PROCEDURE FOR HYPOPLASTIC LEFT HEART

The Norwood procedure is a complex surgical technique classically used to repair hypoplastic left heart syndrome (*see* page 122). Only a basic understanding is required.

This is a three-staged procedure for palliation; it does not correct the underlying problem but leaves a single, univentricular pumping system behind.

The aim of this operation is to have the single ventricle acting as the pump for blood to move around the systemic circulation. The venous return from the body enters the pulmonary vasculature directly, before returning to the heart to go around the body.

Stage I Norwood

This is the initial operation performed in the neonatal period (usually first week of life).

It is a high-risk procedure compared to other forms of cardiac surgery (~80% survival).

The operation involves the following.
➤ Atrial septectomy (removal of all atrial wall, to make one common atria).
➤ Disconnecting the main pulmonary artery (MPA) from the heart and using the residual end of the MPA arising from the right ventricle to fuse to the small ascending aorta making a 'neo-aorta'.
➤ Inserting a shunt into the pulmonary artery to ensure pulmonary blood flow: modified BT shunt (*see* page 82) is a synthetic tube that connects one of the subclavian arteries to the branch PA (Figure 6.37A); a Sano-modification shunt is an alternative to a BT shunt. This is a synthetic tube that is fixed into the RV and joins to the branch PA ('RV-PA conduit') (Figure 6.37B).

By the end of this operation the following will take place.
➤ Blood enters the RV (which is now the systemic ventricle) through the tricuspid valve (note that all blood is mixed together so baby is still cyanotic).
➤ When the RV contracts: blood exits the RV through the neo-aorta

(consisting of the pulmonary valve, and old aorta and synthetic material); blood exits the RV through the Sano shunt (if present) and goes to the lungs for oxygenation; if Sano shunt is not present, as the blood passes up the neo-aorta, a proportion will pass through the BT shunt and go to the lungs.

➤ The blood passes around the body and returns to the common atria through the SVC and IVC.

➤ Blood returns back from the lungs in the pulmonary veins to the common atria.

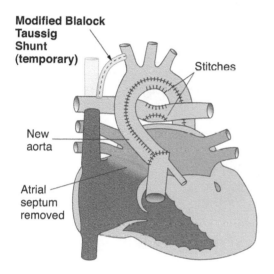

FIGURE 6.37A Stage I Norwood

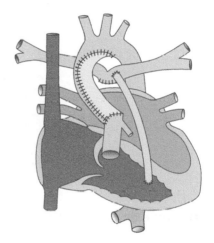

FIGURE 6.37B Stage I Norwood with Sano modification

Stage II Norwood

(Also called: bidirectional Glenn shunt or Hemi-Fontan procedure) (Figure 6.38).

This operation is performed in the first 3 to 6 months of life, when the pulmonary vascular resistance has fallen (often diagnostic catheter performed first).

This operation involves:

➤ removing the BT or Sano shunt

➤ disconnecting the SVC from the RA and connecting it directly to the branch PA.

By the end of this operation the following will occur.

➤ When the RV contracts the blood exits the RV through the neo-aorta, but this time all the blood goes to the systemic circulation (as no shunt left).

➤ Blood returns to the heart:

  ➢ from the body via the IVC to the common atria

  ➢ from the lungs via the pulmonary veins to the common atria.

➤ Blood now directly enters the pulmonary circulation from the head/upper limbs via the SVC directly to the PAs (hence need low PVR so that the SVC can drain passively into the PAs). As a result of this, there is less mixing of oxygenated and deoxygenated blood.

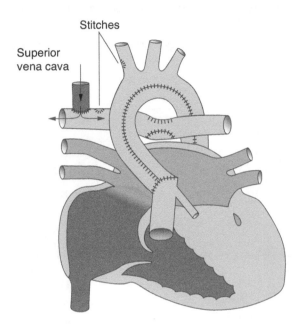

FIGURE 6.38 Stage II Norwood

Stage III Norwood

(Also known as completion of Fontan circulation, or total cavopulmonary connection (TCPC)) (Figure 6.39).

This is the final stage of completing the univentricular system, usually performed around 5 years old, but it can be varied depending on how well the child is coping with Stage II (as children may outgrow the bidirectional Glenn shunt, indicated by falling saturations).

This operation involves removing the IVC from the RA and attaching it to the PAs.

As a result, all the systemic deoxygenated blood returns directly to the pulmonary circulation, bypassing the heart, resulting in no mixing of blood.

The child may have saturations of 100%, although there are variations in surgery.

Importance for general paediatrics

Children undergoing the Norwood procedure, and after it, can deteriorate very rapidly; any symptoms need to be taken seriously.

Two common situations to be aware of are as follows.

1   Respiratory infections (e.g. bronchiolitis) can raise pulmonary vascular resist-
    ance (PVR), so less blood flow occurs from the SVC/IVC to the PAs. The child
    desaturates, possibly with some facial swelling. If severe they may need vent-
    ilating, with the use of pulmonary vasodilators (e.g. nitric oxide).
2   Dehydration (e.g. severe D&V) will result in a reduced intravascular volume.
    This can result in a reduced pressure in the SVC/IVC, so less blood flows into
    the PAs. These children often need IV maintenance fluids.

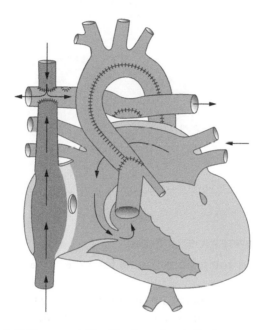

FIGURE 6.39 Stage III Norwood (the Fontan circulation)

Partial anomalous pulmonary venous drainage (PAPVD) – *see under*
  Total anomalous pulmonary venous drainage (TAPVD)
Patau syndrome (trisomy 13) – *see* Syndromes associated with
  cardiac abnormalities
Patent ductus arteriosus (PDA)
Patent foramen ovale – *see under* Atrial septal defect (ASD)
Pericardial effusion
Pericarditis
Persistent pulmonary hypertension of the newborn (PPHN)
Pulmonary arterial hypertension
Pulmonary artery (PA) band
Pulmonary atresia
Pulmonary stenosis (PS)

PATENT DUCTUS ARTERIOSUS (PDA)

Isolated patent ductus arteriosus accounts for 12%–15% of all congenital heart lesions.

The ductus arteriosus connects the pulmonary artery to the descending aorta.

In the fetus, most of the pulmonary blood flows through the ductus arteriosus into the aorta, largely bypassing the non-aerated lung.

In most babies, functional closure of the duct occurs soon after birth.

If the duct fails to close, aortic blood is shunted into the pulmonary artery: a left to right shunt.

Anatomical closure occurs at 1–6 weeks of age.

PDA is more common in girls, 2:1 female:male ratio.

The aortic end of the ductus is just distal to the origin of the left subclavian artery.

It is a common problem in neonatal intensive care units, and is usually as a result of hypoxia and immaturity with normal anatomy. It is often not considered a congenital heart defect in preterm babies.

➤ Significant in the preterm infant due to risk of pulmonary haemorrhage, necrotising enterocolitis and ventilation dependency (and risk of chronic lung disease).

In premature infants most patent ducts will close spontaneously, though some will require pharmacological or surgical intervention.

It is found in association with maternal rubella infection early in pregnancy, where it occurs in combination with other anomalies.

PDA anatomy

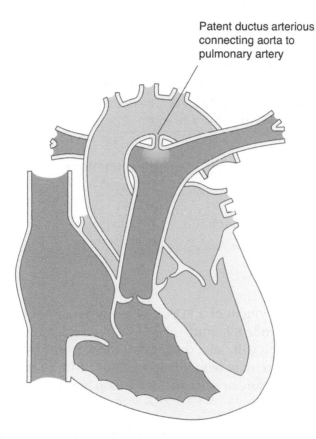

Patent ductus arterious connecting aorta to pulmonary artery

FIGURE 6.40

Pathophysiology

After birth as pulmonary vascular resistance falls, aortic blood is shunted into the pulmonary artery.

The extent of the shunt depends on:

➤ the ratio of pulmonary to systemic vascular resistance
➤ the size of the ductus arteriosus.

With a large PDA the left ventricular, left atrial, pulmonary and right ventricular pressures will be elevated.

Pulmonary arterial pressure may be elevated to systemic levels.

Investigations

Investigation	Description
ECG	Left ventricular and left atrial enlargement
	+/− biventricular hypertrophy if raised main pulmonary artery pressure
Chest X-ray	Cardiomegaly
	Prominent pulmonary artery
	Increased pulmonary vascular markings
Echo	Left to right shunt at the pulmonary artery level
	Must exclude duct-dependent lesions before treating a PDA
Catheter	Normal or increased pressure in the right ventricle and pulmonary artery depending on the size of the shunt

Clinical features

> Bounding pulses
> Active praecordium
> Continuous systolic murmur heard at the left sternal edge
> +/− collapsing pulse

Investigations

> ECG
> CXR
> Echo
> Catheter

Management

Before considering treatment of a PDA, a detailed echo must be carried out to exclude any duct-dependent lesion!

Untreated large ducts will cause congestive cardiac failure (*see* page 84).

In symptomatic preterm or term infants treatment with pharmacological, cardiac catheter device closure or surgical intervention may be required.

Preterm infants
➤ In most preterm infants the patent duct will close spontaneously.
➤ Fluid restriction and diuretics may be tried.
➤ Medical duct closure can be attempted using indomethacin or ibuprofen.

Older children
➤ Spontaneous closure of the duct after infancy is extremely rare.
➤ Device closure of the PDA during cardiac catheterisation is frequently performed.
➤ In some cases, surgical ligation of the PDA may be necessary (e.g. when associated with other cardiac lesions or unusual shape PDA).

PERICARDIAL EFFUSION

Pericardial effusion is a term used to describe increased fluid in the pericardial space around the heart (Figure 6.41). The anatomy of the pericardium is discussed in more detail in Chapter 2.

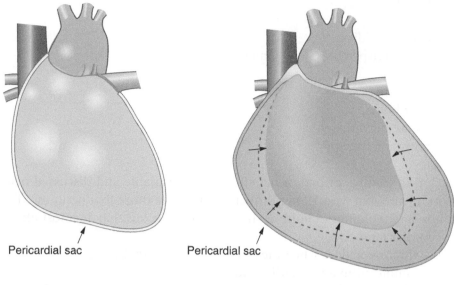

Normal pericardium   Pericardial effusion

FIGURE 6.41 Pericardial effusion

Pericardial effusion is a diagnosis. Although a cause may not always be found, investigations in children should be targeted to try to find one.

Causes of pericardial effusions include the following.
➤ Idiopathic
➤ Infectious (acute pericarditis is the commonest cause):
  ➤ viral (e.g. coxsackie virus, echovirus, adenovirus, Epstein-Barr virus, mumps)
  ➤ bacterial (e.g. *Streptococcus, Pneumococcus, Staphylococcus*)
  ➤ don't forget rare infections such as TB, fungal infections and parasites in those with foreign travel or immunocompromised children.
➤ Cardiac disease
  ➤ pericarditis
  ➤ aortic dissection
  ➤ cardiomyopathy
  ➤ myocarditis.
➤ Rheumatic fever
➤ Trauma
  ➤ post-cardiac surgery
  ➤ thoracic trauma.
➤ Rheumatological
  ➤ systemic lupus erythematosus
  ➤ familial Mediterranean fever
  ➤ rheumatoid arthritis.

➤ Metabolic
  ➢ uraemia
  ➢ hypothyroidism
  ➢ familial hypercholesterolaemia.
➤ Malignancy
  ➢ leukaemia
  ➢ lymphoma
  ➢ metastatic disease
  ➢ post-radiotherapy.

The clinical features of pericardial effusions are variable and discussed below. The most worrying types of pericardial effusions are those that occur rapidly or result in large volumes of fluid, as these are the effusions that are most likely to cause cardiac tamponade.

Cardiac tamponade is when the heart is under external compression.
➤ For example, from a pericardial effusion.
➤ This causes a restriction in ventricular filling, with a subsequent reduction in cardiac output and therefore haemodynamic compromise.
➤ This is a medical emergency and can be fatal without treatment.
➤ It is one of the reversible causes of cardiac arrest.

Management includes the following.
➤ Treating the underlying cause.
➤ Emergency pericardiocentesis if true cardiac tamponade.
➤ Pericardiocentesis and pericardial drain if large, but no tamponade.
➤ Careful monitoring and observation if small – moderate effusion with no haemodynamic compromise.
➤ Rarely, surgical management is required to drain the effusion or treat certain underlying causes.

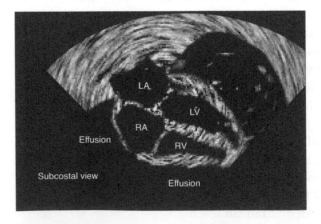

FIGURE 6.42 Pericardial effusion on echocardiography

Clinical features

> Asymptomatic
> Features suggestive of an underlying cause (e.g. pericarditis, SLE, malignancy)
> Often non-specific in effusions
> ✓ Chest pain (eased by sitting forward)
> ✓ Shortness of breath
> ✓ Dizziness
> ✓ Cough
> In cardiac tamponade:
> ✓ Unwell, shocked with low cardiac output
> ✓ Tachycardia and tachypnoea
> ✓ Decrease in BP with inspiration (pulsus paradoxus)
> ✓ Beck's Triad
> 1 Hypotension
> 2 Muffled heart sounds
> 3 Raised JVP (difficult in children)

Investigations

1 CXR may show an increased cardiothoracic ratio, but it will not determine if this is due to cardiomegaly or effusion.
2 ECG may show low voltage QRS complexes due to the effusion. It may also demonstrate the typical changes seen with pericarditis.
3 Echo will show fluid in the pericardial space (Figure 6.42), as well assess for haemodynamic compromise associated with cardiac tamponade.
4 Blood investigations should be taken to asses for a cause based on the list given above (e.g. urea, viral titres, blood cultures, auto-antibodies etc.).

PERICARDITIS

Inflammation of the pericardium.

Children usually present with a retrosternal chest pain.

The pain varies with respiration and position and is often relieved by sitting forward.

The pericardium becomes acutely inflamed with an infiltration of leucocytes with subsequent pericardial vascularisation.

Some 20%–80% of cases are idiopathic with a large number of these likely due to undiagnosed viral infections.

Accumulation of fluid may lead to a pericardial effusion with subsequent cardiac tamponade.

Idiopathic and viral pericarditis usually have a self-limiting cause.

Prognosis depends upon the aetiology and the presence of an effusion.

Management is supportive with anti-inflammatory drugs, treatment of the underlying cause and surgical drainage of large effusions.

Anatomy

The pericardium is composed of two layers:
➤ parietal pericardium – outer fibrous layer
➤ visceral pericardium – an inner serous, single membrane layer.

The pericardium forms a protective barrier against the spread of infection and inflammation from adjacent structures.

Causative organisms/factors

Viral	Coxsackie
	Enterovirus
Bacterial	*Staphylococcus aureus*
	Streptococcal pneumonia
	Tuberculosis
Fungal	Histoplasma
	Candida
	Aspergillus
Other	SLE
	Rheumatic fever
	Rheumatoid arthritis
	Sarcoidosis
	Juvenile idiopathic arthritis (JIA)
	Uraemia
	Post irradiation
	Hypothyroidism
	Trauma
	Malignancy

ECG changes seen in acute pericarditis

➤ ST elevation
➤ T-wave inversion
➤ Saddle or concave elevation (with the exception of aVR).

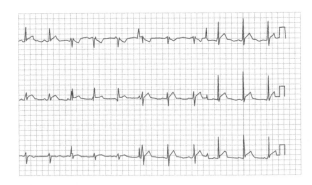

FIGURE 6.43 ECG of pericarditis

Pulsus paradoxus: increase in the normal physiological fall in pulse pressure on inspiration. During inspiration systolic pressure decreases by 20 mmHg.

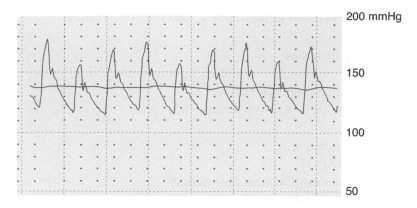

FIGURE 6.44 Graphical representation of pulsus paradoxus (an increase in the normal physiological fall in pulse pressure on inspiration)

Clinical features
> Fever
> Tachycardia
> Pericardial friction rub
> Raised JVP
> Hyper/hypotension
> Pulsus paradoxus
> Features of underlying condition

Investigations
> FBC
> CRP, ESR
> Blood culture
> CXR
> ECG
> Echo

PERSISTENT PULMONARY HYPERTENSION OF THE NEWBORN (PPHN)

Persistent pulmonary hypertension of the newborn involves failure of the normal transitional circulatory changes to occur after birth from placental to pulmonary respiration (*see* page 15).

It is characterised by a marked pulmonary hypertension leading to hypoxaemia and right to left shunting of blood, causing cyanosis.

Usually, soon after birth there is a decrease in pulmonary vascular resistance and an increase in pulmonary blood flow. In some newborns these normal circulatory changes do not occur after birth, resulting in PPHN.

It is estimated to occur in approximately 2 in 1000 live born term babies.

As a result of high pulmonary vascular resistance there is right to left shunting at both atrial and ductal levels, as the pulmonary blood pressure often exceeds systemic blood pressure.

It sometimes occurs as a primary disorder; however, it more frequently arises in association with:
➤ respiratory distress syndrome
➤ septicaemia
➤ birth asphyxia
➤ meconium aspiration.

Causes of a delayed fall in pulmonary vascular resistance:

➤ Respiratory:
  ➢ meconium aspiration
  ➢ pneumonia
  ➢ congenital diaphragmatic hernia
  ➢ obstructed middle or lower airway.
➤ Cardiac:
  ➢ pulmonary stenosis
  ➢ obstructed TAPVD
  ➢ left ventricular outflow tract obstruction
  ➢ left ventricular dysfunction
  ➢ AVSD
  ➢ coronary arteriovenous fistula
  ➢ cerebral ateriovenous malformation
  ➢ Ebstein's anomaly
  ➢ Ductal closure *in utero.*
➤ Other:
  ➢ sepsis
  ➢ idiopathic PPHN (primary disorder).

Pulmonary arterial pressure (P) is the product of pulmonary vascular resistance (R) and pulmonary blood flow (F):

$$P = R \times F$$

The key underlying pathophysiology is the raised pulmonary vascular resistance.

Pulmonary vasoconstriction and hypertension following hypoxaemia can result in right to left shunting.

It is vital that PPHN is distinguished from cyanotic heart disease; this can be difficult.

Investigations

Investigation	Description
Arterial blood gases (ABG)	Hypercapnia – if profound his should be treated actively
	Hypoxia
CXR	Pulmonary oligaemia
Echo	Exclude structural disease
	Features of PPHN include significant tricuspid regurgitation, poor right ventricular function and the interventricular septum is pushed towards the left (suggesting RV pressures are higher than LV pressures)
Four-limb blood pressure	May be normal or hypotensive
Oxygen saturations	Lower in feet than upper limbs

Management

Mechanical ventilation:
➤ maintain normal acid–base balance with $PaCo_2$ 3–4 kPa.

Pulmonary vasodilators:
➤ oxygen (targeting normal saturations once structural heart disease is excluded)
➤ inhaled nitric oxide.

Extracorporeal membrane oxygenation:
➤ this is effective and is indicated for severe cases
➤ *see* page 106.

PULMONARY ARTERIAL HYPERTENSION

Pulmonary hypertension is a clinical syndrome characterised by an increased resistance in the right side of the heart, in the absence of raised left-sided pressures.

Pulmonary hypertension is defined by a mean pulmonary artery pressure of more than 25 mmHg at rest or more than 30 mmHg during exercise.

Pathophysiology

Pulmonary hypertension is associated with obstruction of the pulmonary vascular bed due to hyperplasia of the muscular and elastic tissues.

This leads to the pulmonary vasculature of the lungs having an increased amount of muscle in the vessel walls.

When the ratio of pulmonary to systemic vascular resistance exceeds 0.7, the degree of pulmonary vascular disease is considered to be irreversible.

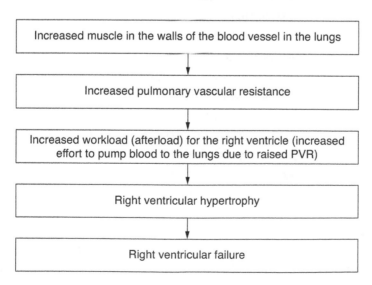

FIGURE 6.45 Understanding the pathophysiology of pulmonary hypertension

Aetiology

1 Congenital heart disease:
   - left–right shunt: VSD, PDA
   - TAPVD
   - truncus arteriosus
   - TGA
   - left ventricular outflow obstruction
   - pulmonary vein stenosis or veno-occlusive disease
   - Eisenmenger syndrome (*see* page 106).
2 Pulmonary vascular disease:
   - primary idiopathic pulmonary arterial hypertension
   - persistent pulmonary hypertension of the newborn
   - systemic lupus erythematosus.
3 Chronic lung disease:
   - airways obstruction: chronic asthma, adenoidal/tonsillar hypertrophy
   - restrictive disorders: kyphoscoliosis
   - parenchymal disorders: cystic fibrosis.
4 Other:
   - neuromuscular disorders
   - high altitude
   - familial.

INVESTIGATIONS

Investigation	Description
ECG	Right axis deviation
	Right ventricular hypertrophy
	Right atrial hypertrophy
CXR	Increased cardiac shadow
	Enlarged pulmonary trunk
	Congested proximal pulmonary arteries
Echo	Rule out congenital heart disease
	Tricuspid regurgitation
	Enlarged right ventricle with reduced RV function
	Estimated right ventricular pressure raised
Catheter	Increased right-sided pressures
	Pulmonary artery hypertension

Management

Needs to be treated aggressively. A national Paediatric UK Pulmonary Arterial Hypertension service exists, led by Great Ormond Street Hospital, London.

Early surgical intervention and prevention of any underlying causative disease is essential.

Heart-lung transplant may be considered.

Medical treatment may slow progression and offer symptomatic relief:

➤ oxygen
➤ inhaled nitric oxide
➤ diuretics
➤ sildenafil
➤ bosentan
➤ prostacyclin.

Clinical features

❯ Fatigue
❯ Effort intolerance
❯ Precordial chest pain
❯ Syncope
❯ Cyanosis
❯ Cold peripheries
❯ Signs of right-sided heart failure:
  ✓ Raised JVP
  ✓ Oedema
  ✓ Hepatomegaly
  ✓ Right ventricular heave
❯ Progressive dyspnoea
❯ Haemoptysis
❯ Loud second heart sound

Investigations

❯ ECG
❯ CXR
❯ Echo
❯ Exercise test
❯ Cardiac catheterisation

PULMONARY ARTERY (PA) BAND

Pulmonary artery band is a surgical procedure used to reduce pulmonary blood flow.

This is important to prevent damage to the pulmonary vascular bed (and potential pulmonary hypertension) by limiting the volume of blood that can reach the pulmonary circulation.

This is a palliative procedure; it does not correct the underlying congenital heart defect. Further surgery will be needed later to remove the PA band and operate on the original defect.

This operation is much less common, as many defects can be repaired as a primary operation, reducing the need for palliative surgery. It is often used in very small babies or in situations where it is not possible to repair the heart in one operation.

The PA band is a non-bypass operation, performed through a lateral thoracotomy incision.

The PA band is placed usually on the main pulmonary artery, thus creating a 'pulmonary stenosis' and preventing excessive blood entering the branch pulmonary arteries (Figure 6.46). Occasionally, two PA bands can be inserted, one on each branch PA.

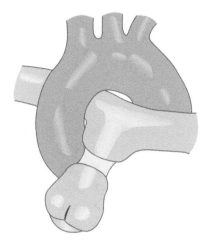

FIGURE 6.46 A PA band placed on the main pulmonary artery

Possible situations when the PA band has been used due to high pulmonary blood flow include:
➤ large or multiple ventricular septal defect with high left to right shunting
➤ unbalanced atrioventricular septal defects (with small left ventricle)
➤ single ventricle systems with high pulmonary blood flow (e.g. double inlet left ventricle).

The PA band has some problems, as follows.
➤ It is difficult in a neonate to know how tight to place the band. Balancing pulmonary and systemic circulations is difficult.
➤ As the child grows the PA band will not, and so get tighter. This will means less pulmonary blood flow and so the child will become cyanotic.
➤ A second operation will be required to remove the PA band.
➤ The PA band may leave behind damage to the pulmonary artery.

PULMONARY ATRESIA (PA)
Pulmonary atresia is a cyanotic congenital heart defect where there is absence of opening in the right ventricular outflow tract (i.e. no pulmonary valve or segment of the main pulmonary artery).

This means that there is a reduction in pulmonary blood flow, resulting in cyanosis.

Pulmonary blood flow will depend on the degree of shunting through:
➤ patent ductus arteriosus

➤ patent foramen ovale

➤ associated lesions such as a ventricular septal defect.

PA can often be considered as a duct-dependent circulation (*see* page 101), especially if there is no associated VSD.

Two types of PA are recognised:

1   PA with VSD (PA-VSD) – Figure 6.47A

2   PA with intact interventricular septum (PA-IVS) – Figure 6.47B.

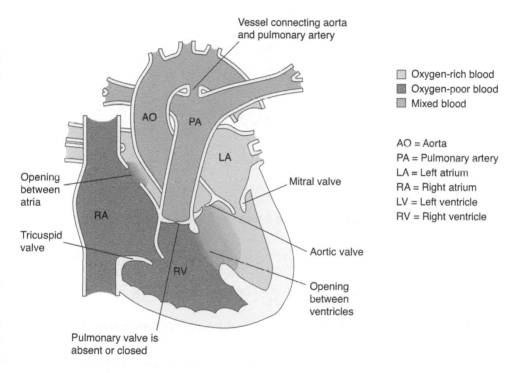

FIGURE 6.47A Pulmonary atresia with ventricular septal defect (PA-VSD)

PA with VSD (Figure 6.47A)

➤ Most common type of pulmonary atresia.

➤ The VSD provides an extra level of shunting of blood from the right to left side (to get blood to the aorta and PDA).

➤ The spectrum of PA-VSD can vary and can include Fallot's type pulmonary atresia – RVH, VSD, overriding aorta and pulmonary atresia (rather than RV outflow obstruction due to stenosis).

PA with IVS (Figure 6.47B)

➤ Less common that PA with VSD.

➤ Because there is no VSD, less shunting of blood occurs and so the child is often cyanosed and duct-dependent.

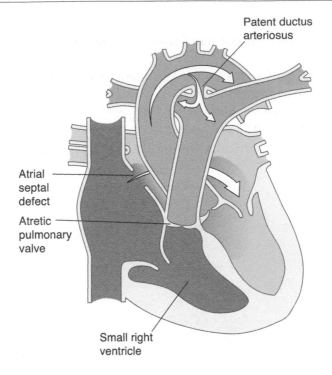

FIGURE 6.47B Pulmonary atresia with intact ventricular septum (PA-IVS)

➤ The shunting through the PFO has to be right to left (to get blood to the aorta and PDA).
➤ The shunting through the PDA has to be left to right (to get blood to the lungs).
➤ The right ventricle is often hypoplastic, which affects longer term treatment.

PA may be diagnosed in the antenatal period. If not, it usually presents in the neonatal period with cyanosis.

PA can also have major aortopulmonary collateral arteries (MAPCAs) associated with the other defects. These are vessels that develop in fetal life from the aorta to provide blood supply to the pulmonary circulation, when the normal pulmonary artery is underdeveloped.

PA is associated with:
➤ DiGeorge syndrome (22q11 microdeletion)
➤ velocardiofacial syndrome.

Management is as follows.
➤ Initial resuscitation and stabilisation (as per APLS and NLS protocols).
➤ Obtain two good IV access points and commence prostaglandin treatment.
➤ Arrange transfer to a paediatric cardiology unit.

➤ Further management is initially aimed at increasing pulmonary blood flow:
  ➤ balloon atrial septostomy (*see* page 171) to increase right to left flow through the PFO
  ➤ surgical shunt (e.g. BT shunt).
➤ If the RV is of good size, full corrective surgery can be undertaken at a later date.
➤ If the RV is hypoplastic, a single ventricle repair may be needed.

Clinical features

> Antenatal diagnosis
> Neonatal cyanosis (worsening as duct closes)
> Murmur of VSD if present
> Dysmorphism if associated with a syndrome

Investigations

1 ECG can be normal. It may show right atrial enlargement (P-pulmonale) and LV dominance if the RV is small.
2 CXR can show cardiomegaly and reduced pulmonary vascular markings.
3 Echo will confirm the diagnosis and associated defects.
4 Diagnostic cardiac catheter may be indicated to help identify complex anatomy (e.g. MAPCAs).
5 FISH for 22q11 microdeletion.

PULMONARY STENOSIS (PS)

Pulmonary stenosis accounts for 8% of congenital heart lesions.
Most children with pulmonary valve stenosis are asymptomatic but age of presentation can vary.
➤ A neonate with critical pulmonary stenosis has a duct-dependent lesion and will present within the few days of life due to reduced pulmonary blood flow.
➤ A mild form may go undetected for years.

The right ventricular wall becomes increasingly hypertrophied.
➤ Increased resistance to right ventricular ejection is the underlying abnormality.

The obstruction can be at three levels: supravalvular, valvular or subvalvular.
➤ The most common anatomical site for the stenotic lesion is the actual valve itself.
➤ You can also get peripheral branch pulmonary artery stenosis, which is often a normal finding in neonates.

Infundibular hypertrophy is a common accompanying finding in pulmonary stenosis.

Anatomy of pulmonary valve stenosis

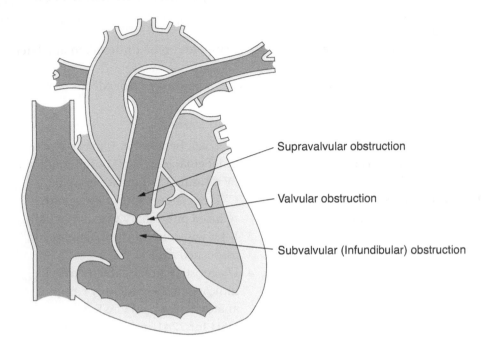

Supravalvular obstruction

Valvular obstruction

Subvalvular (Infundibular) obstruction

FIGURE 6.48

Stenosis at the pulmonary valve level is associated with:
➤ Noonan syndrome
➤ congenital rubella syndrome
➤ Williams syndrome
➤ Alagille syndrome.

Stenosis at the supravalvular level is associated with:
➤ Williams syndrome
➤ DiGeorge syndrome
➤ Alagille syndrome
➤ congenital rubella syndrome
➤ Noonan syndrome.

Obstruction to the right ventricular outflow tract forms part of the tetralogy of Fallot (usually a mix of subvalvular and valvular pulmonary stenosis).

Investigations

Investigation	Description
ECG	Right ventricular hypertrophy for age
CXR	Poststenotic dilatation of the main pulmonary artery
	Cardiomegaly
Echo	Diagnostic of pulmonary stenosis and associated lesions
	Assessment of RV function and any RV hypertrophy
Catheter	The right ventricular systolic pressure can exceed the systemic pressure in severe cases

Management

Surgery is indicated when the transvalvular gradient crosses approximately 50 mmHg: either valve replacement or a surgical valvotomy.

Balloon dilatation performed during cardiac catheterisation is used to relieve the obstruction in some cases (especially neonatal critical pulmonary stenosis).

Critical pulmonary stenosis in the neonate may need prostaglandin until definitive surgery, following a similar initial management plan to pulmonary atresia (*see* page 162).

Clinical features

> Usually asymptomatic
> Ejection systolic murmur – best heard in the second and third upper left intercostal spaces and radiates to the back
> Prolonged right ventricular impulse with delayed pulmonary valve closure
> Mild fatigue
> Dyspnoea
> Cyanosis
> Congestive heart failure

Investigations

> CXR
> ECG
> Echo
> Catheter

QT PROLONGATION (LONG QT SYNDROME)

The QT interval is the period of time taken for ventricular depolarisation and repolarisation to occur (i.e. ventricular contraction then relaxation).

The QT interval needs to vary with heart rates to allow the ventricles to contract quicker if needed. We therefore 'correct' the QT value for heart rate using Bazett's formula. This is discussed in more detail in Chapter 4.

When the QT is prolonged you can get depolarisation occurring before the ventricles repolarise – this leads to arrhythmias (often a polymorphic ventricular tachycardia known as torsades de pointes, followed by ventricular fibrillation in some cases). This clinically presents with syncope or sudden cardiac death.

Typically, a QTc of over 440 ms is called prolonged, although neonates and females can have a slightly higher value. A QTc of over 480 ms is significant in all groups.

A prolonged QT in the paediatric practise can be congenital long QT syndrome (LQTS) (with a genetic mutation found in up to 70% of cases) or acquired (a pathological increase in the QT interval in response to a stimuli).

Causes of acquired prolonged QT include:
➤ drug exposure
➤ many including certain antibiotics, anti-arrhythmics, chemotherapeutic agents, antiemetics, antipsychotics – please consult appropriate drug literature for further information
➤ electrolyte imbalance
➤ hypokalaemia, hypocalcaemia and hypomagnesaemia
➤ post-cardiac surgery
➤ head injury
➤ hypothermia
➤ acute carditis.

As mentioned, gene testing is useful in congenital LQTS with many genes identified causing different types of LQTS. The genetic testing is useful in that the genotype present can be used to screen other family members, but also can predict the phenotype of the patient.
➤ LQT1 (caused by mutation in KCNQ1 gene):
  ➢ high frequency of syncope on exercise (especially swimming)
  ➢ less sudden cardiac death than the others.

➤ LQT2 (caused by mutation in KCNH2 gene):
  ➢ equally triggered by exercise and sleep, but specifically associated with auditory stimuli (e.g. alarm clock, mobile phones, sudden noise)
➤ LQT3 (caused by mutation in SCN5A gene)
  ➢ often not exercise triggered; usually triggered by sleep/rest.

Jervell and Lange–Nielsen syndrome is the association of LQTS with sensorineural hearing loss.

LQTS is a disease of young people. Half of the cases have their first event by the age of 18; almost all by the age of 40 years old. It can present in neonates.

The exact incidence is unknown, but some reports suggest 1 in 5000 people.

A good clinical history is important when you suspect long QT syndrome and must include:
➤ syncope (especially in response to a 'stress' which can include exercise, sudden auditory stimulus, sleep, strong emotions) – a detailed history must be taken.
➤ family history of sudden cardiac death
➤ family history of known LQTS
➤ 'seizures' (can represent hypoxia from the VT, especially if sleep triggered)
➤ sensorineural hearing loss
➤ general lifestyle of the child (important for management planning).

Management of long QT needs to be undertaken carefully, but includes the following.
➤ Screening of all the family members.
➤ Lifestyle advice (e.g. removing risk factors, gradual increase and decrease in exercise, avoid sudden stresses).
➤ Treat any underlying causes.
➤ β-blockers:
  ➢ e.g. nadolol, atenolol or propranolol
  ➢ provide protective effect against syncope/arrhythmia but do not return QTc to normal
  ➢ monitor effect of treatment by ensuring heart rate is suitably β-blocked.
➤ Pacemaker insertion.
➤ Implantable cardioverter defibrillator (ICD):
  ➢ only used in those with high risk of sudden cardiac death.

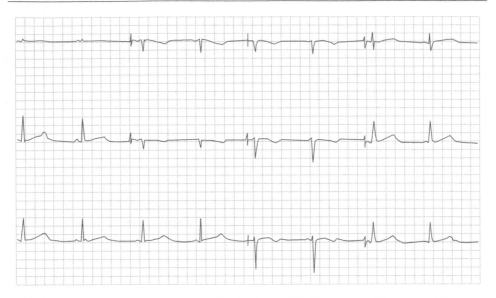

FIGURE 6.49 An example of an ECG with long QT. (Note the wide-based T waves)

Clinical features

> Asymptomatic
> Found on screening due to other family members with the disease
> Family history of sudden cardiac death
> Family history of long QT
> Sensorineural deafness
> Syncope
  ✓ Especially on exercise, sudden noise or emotional stress
  ✓ May have 'jerking of limbs' due to hypoxia
> Normal cardiovascular examination (although may be borderline bradycardic in some cases)

Investigations

1 12-lead ECG may show a long QTc (may be normal or borderline in a few cases) or T-wave abnormalities (e.g. biphasic, wide based, variable morphology in same ECG) or a low heart rate for age (Figure 6.49).
2 Holter monitor/24-hour tape may show periods of arrhythmia (usually polymorphic VT) or failure of QT interval to shorten during exercise.
3 Exercise testing can demonstrate failure of the QT interval to shorten during exercise (useful if strongly suspicious on history but normal ECG) and can assess child is suitable β-blocked as part of treatment.
4 Genetic testing (after discussion with genetics team).
5 Electrolytes.

Rashkind procedure (balloon atrial septostomy)
Rastelli procedure
Rheumatic fever
Romano–Ward syndrome – *see* Syndromes associated with cardiac
   abnormalities

RASHKIND PROCEDURE (BALLOON ATRIAL SEPTOSTOMY)

The Rashkind procedure is more often referred to as a balloon atrial septostomy.
It is an example of an interventional cardiac catheterisation procedure.

The aim of the procedure is to create a larger opening in the atrial septum to increase the mixing of blood between the left and right circulations, in situations where the neonate has inadequate mixing of circulations and is severely cyanotic. It is only a temporary measure until cardiac surgery.

Examples of when a balloon atrial septostomy may be indicated include:
➤ transposition of the great arteries (commonest indication)
➤ congenital heart defects with reduced mixing (e.g. pulmonary atresia with intact septum or hypoplastic left heart syndrome)
➤ severe pulmonary hypertension (rarely done).

The procedure involves the following.
➤ Passing a catheter wire into the right atrium, either via the femoral or umbilical vein.
➤ The catheter is then guided through the foramen ovale into the left atria.
➤ The balloon on the end of the catheter is inflated, while in the left atria.
➤ The balloon is then pulled across the foramen ovale into the right atria again, thus widening the foramen ovale and allowing more mixing of blood.
➤ The balloon is pulled as many times as is needed to create a large enough communication between the atria to allow unrestricted mixing of blood.

Figure 6.50 displays the Rashkind procedure.

RASTELLI PROCEDURE

The Rastelli procedure is a surgical technique initially used to repair a heart with three defects (Figure 6.51):
1 Transposition of the great arteries (TGA)

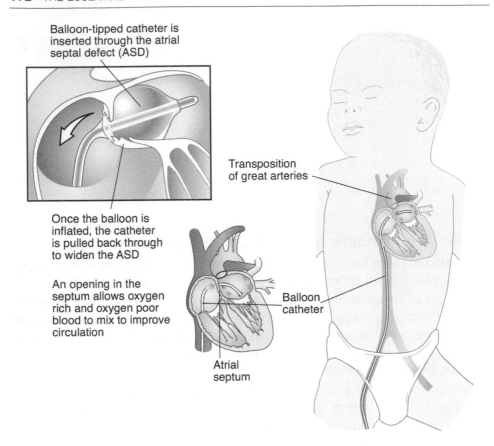

Balloon-tipped catheter is inserted through the atrial septal defect (ASD)

Transposition of great arteries

Once the balloon is inflated, the catheter is pulled back through to widen the ASD

An opening in the septum allows oxygen rich and oxygen poor blood to mix to improve circulation

Balloon catheter

Atrial septum

FIGURE 6.50 Balloon atrial septostomy (Rashkind procedure)

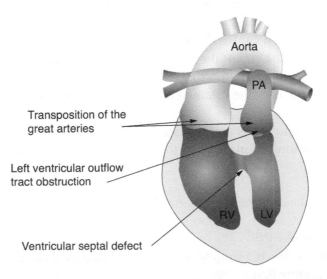

Aorta

PA

Transposition of the great arteries

Left ventricular outflow tract obstruction

RV LV

Ventricular septal defect

FIGURE 6.51 The combination of defects suitable for a Rastelli procedure

2 Ventricular septal defect (VSD)

3 A form of left ventricular outflow tract obstruction (i.e. pulmonary stenosis).

This operation is performed on cardiopulmonary bypass and involves a midline sternotomy.

The operation involves:

➤ using a patch to:
  ➣ direct the blood from the left ventricle to the aorta (which was arising from the right ventricle)
  ➣ close the VSD at the same time
➤ using a channel (conduit) from the right ventricle to the pulmonary artery (which was arising from the left ventricle).

Figure 6.52 demonstrates the procedure.

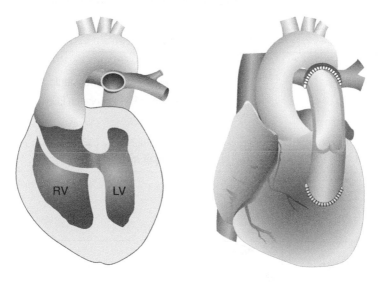

FIGURE 6.52 The appearance of a Rastelli procedure (left – interior; right – exterior)

The Rastelli procedure with some modifications has more recently been used for other defects (e.g. double outlet right ventricle) with the VSD and right ventricle outflow tract (RVOT) obstruction.

RHEUMATIC FEVER

The incidence of rheumatic fever and rheumatic heart disease has decreased in the UK over the last 50 years.

Worldwide it remains the most common cause of acquired heart disease in children.

Rheumatic fever is a serious systemic illness that occurs in adults and children following infection with group A beta haemolytic streptococci, usually in the form of pharyngitis.

Group A streptococci elicit an acute inflammatory response.

After a latent period of 2–6 weeks following a sore throat, individuals usually present with persistent fever, malaise and polyarthralgia.

Development of a pancarditis is common, with approximately 50% of those affected suffering from cardiac damage.

Management is largely supportive with the addition of high-dose aspirin to suppress the ongoing inflammatory response. Steroids are used in resistant cases.

Penicillin or erythromycin in allergic cases is used daily, with recent studies suggesting lifelong prophylaxis once the acute phase has resolved.

Jones criteria for the diagnosis of rheumatic fever

Required are two major *or* one major plus two minor criteria. In addition there must be supporting evidence of preceding streptococcal infection.

Major	Minor
Polyarthritis	Fever
Carditis	Raised acute phase reactants: CRP, ESR
Sydenham's chorea	Prolonged P-R interval on ECG
Erythema marginatum	Leucocytosis
Subcutaneous nodules	Polyarthralgia
	History of rheumatic fever

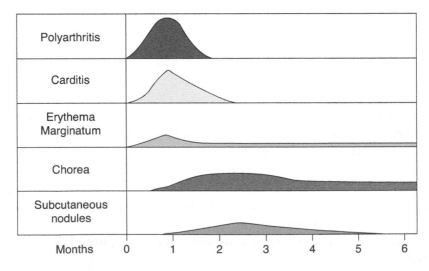

FIGURE 6.53 Clinical manifestations of acute rheumatic fever

Differential diagnoses:

➤ Kawasaki disease
➤ Lyme disease
➤ juvenile idiopathic arthritis
➤ juvenile onset Parkinson's disease
➤ acute lymphocytic leukaemia
➤ systemic lupus erythematosus.

Cardiac complications:

➤ pancarditis
➤ myocarditis
➤ endocarditis
➤ pericarditis
➤ aortic and mitral valve regurgitation
➤ atrial fibrillation (chronic)
➤ congestive heart failure
➤ tricuspid valve deformity.

Chronic rheumatic heart disease

Severe scarring of the mitral and aortic valve occurs months to years after the first presentation of rheumatic fever. Rarely, the pulmonary valve is affected.

Occurs from residual and progressive valve damage. Can lead to chronic severe mitral and aortic valve damage (especially mitral stenosis) and atrial enlargement.

Clinical features	Investigations
❯ Fever	❯ FBC
❯ Polyarthritis: medium-large joints commonly affected	❯ Blood culture CRP, ESR ASOT
❯ Maculopapular rash	❯ Throat swab
❯ Involuntary movements	❯ ECG
❯ Painless hard nodules on extensor surfaces	❯ Echo
❯ New cardiac murmur	❯ CXR
❯ Tachycardia	

Senning procedure – *see under* Mustard procedure
Supraventricular tachycardia (SVT)
Syncope
Syndromes associated with cardiac abnormalities:
- Alagille syndrome
- CHARGE association
- DiGeorge syndrome
- Down syndrome
- Edwards syndrome (Trisomy 18)
- Ehlers–Danlos syndrome
- Goldenhar syndrome
- Holt–Oram syndrome
- Jervell and Lange–Nielsen syndrome
- Klippel–Feil sequence
- Leopard syndrome
- Marfan syndrome
- Noonan syndrome
- Patau syndrome (trisomy 13)
- Romano–Ward syndrome
- Treacher–Collins syndrome
- Tuberous sclerosis
- Turner syndrome
- VACTERL association
- Williams syndrome

SUPRAVENTRICULAR TACHYCARDIA (SVT)

Supraventricular tachycardia is a term used to describe an arrhythmia causing a tachycardia that originates from outside the ventricles (i.e. SA node, atria or AV node).

SVT is the most common paediatric arrhythmia seen.

SVT is a very non-specific term and not a specific diagnosis.

There are many types of SVT. It is important to try to identify the type as this predicts the future of the SVT and will guide management. Seek paediatric cardiology help for this.

Key types of SVT include:
➤ atrioventricular re-entry tachycardia (AVRT)
➤ atrioventricular nodal re-entry tachycardia (AVNRT)
➤ focal atrial tachycardia

➤ permanent junctional re-entry tachycardia (PJRT)
➤ any many more.

It is out of the scope of this book to consider these in more detail. We will now consider SVT as a general concept.

SVT can present in a number of ways from heart failure and cardiovascular compromise in a neonate, to palpitations in the teenager (*see* below).

An ECG should be obtained while in SVT, during cardioversion and after the cardioversion. All will give vital information to help distinguish the type of SVT and subsequent management.

The ECG in SVT will often show (Figure 6.54):

➤ tachycardia (often greater than 220 bpm, but can be as low as 180 bpm)
➤ narrow complex QRS (in certain situations can be wide, if bundle branch block present)
➤ difficult to see P waves (may be masked in other waves)
➤ if P waves are visible may be inverted in II, III and aVF
➤ no beat to beat variation in rate (i.e. fixed RR intervals).

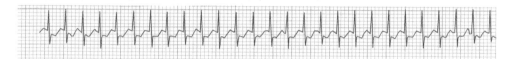

FIGURE 6.54 SVT in a neonate

Adenosine acts as both an investigation and sometimes management of SVT as it blocks the AV node and will either unmask atrial arrhythmias (Figure 6.55A) which can then guide specific treatment, or it may even terminate the SVT (Figure 6.55B).

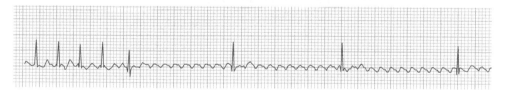

FIGURE 6.55A SVT in a neonate, unmasking atrial flutter with adenosine administration

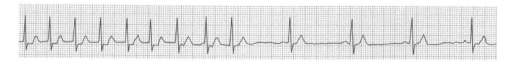

FIGURE 6.55B SVT in an older child, converting to sinus rhythm with adenosine administration

The management of SVT involves terminating the tachycardia. For the SVT management algorithm *see Advanced Paediatric Life Support: The Practical Approach (APLS)*, 5th Edition (Wiley-Blackwell; 2011).

In summary, if the child is haemodynamically stable then vagal manoeuvres can be attempted while IV access is obtained. IV adenosine should then be given, with increasing doses until an affect is seen (either termination of the SVT or unmasking the underlying rhythm). If the child is haemodynamically unstable, you may need urgent DC cardioversion.

Vagal manoeuvres:
➤ Valsalva (e.g. asking older child to blow into the syringe to try to 'blow out the plunger').
➤ Carotid sinus massage (only one side and in older children).
➤ Application of an ice pack to the face (only for 5 seconds, and wrap the rest of the baby first).

As mentioned, each SVT has a specific management. The important one to remember is neonatal atrial flutter is often highly drug resistant and DC cardioversion is the main treatment.

The prognosis of SVT is variable depending on the age of the child, number of previous episodes of SVT and the sub-group of SVT.

Infants often need only one year of prophylactic medication before having all treatment stopped.

Older children are more likely to need further intervention (e.g. ongoing anti-arrhythmic treatment or radiofrequency catheter ablation).

It can be difficult to distinguish between SVT and sinus tachycardia. Table 6.6 summarises some of the key differences that may help distinguish the two.

TABLE 6.6 Distinguishing SVT from sinus tachycardia

	SVT	Sinus tachycardia
History	Previously well	Preceding systemic illness or trauma
	Sudden onset	
Heart rate	Usually greater than 220 bpm	Rarely greater than 220 bpm
	Abrupt changes in heart rate seen	Gradual changes in heart rate
	Responds well to adenosine or Valsalva manoeuvres	Responds to non-cardiac treatments (e.g. fluid, antipyretics)
ECG findings	No beat to beat variability	Beat to beat variability
	Absent P waves *or*	Upright P waves in II, III and aVF
	Inverted P waves in II, III and aVF	
Response to adenosine	If good doses given, may terminate SVT	May have no response, but can sometimes slow down before speeding up again
	Underlying problems (e.g. atrial flutter) may be seen	

Clinical features

> Asymptomatic
> Neonatal heart failure/shock
> Palpitations
  ✓ Sudden onset
  ✓ Sudden termination
  ✓ Rapid and regular
> Syncope
> Dizziness
> Chest pain
> Heart rate usually greater than 220 bpm
> Evidence of haemodynamic compromise

Investigations

1 ECG when in SVT will likely show a narrow complex QRS, with a heart rate greater than 220 bpm and difficult to see P waves. When in sinus rhythm the ECG may be normal, or may show evidence of Wolff–Parkinson–White syndrome. The response to adenosine may show the underlying cause or act as a drug cardioversion.

2 Twenty-four-hour tape or Cardiomemo may help you obtain an idea of how frequent are self-limiting runs of SVT.

SYNCOPE

Syncope is a transient loss of consciousness and postural tone that occurs secondary to transient cerebral anoxia due to cerebral hypoperfusion.

There is a drop in systemic blood pressure which may be of gradual onset or sudden.

The underlying aetiology appears to be a reflex vascular phenomenon which leads to a transient decrease in the oxygen supply to cerebral neurons.

The child will usually complain of feeling dizzy, lightheaded, hot and nauseous prior to collapsing.

The child may also have hypoxic seizures, leading people incorrectly to the diagnosis of epilepsy.

There is no post-ictal phase though the child may feel weak and nauseous.

The diagnosis can usually be made from the history and confirmed with minimal investigations. It is important to recognise serious causes of syncope, although most are benign.

The following features suggest a sinister cause for the syncope:

➤ exercise-induced syncope
➤ syncope when swimming
➤ syncope associated with sudden emotions (e.g. fright, excitement, sudden noise)
➤ sudden unexplained collapse with no obvious trigger to suggest vasovagal syncope
➤ family history of sudden cardiac death or known cardiac defect (e.g. HOCM, long QT)
➤ any abnormalities on cardiovascular examination
➤ any abnormalities on the 12-lead ECG.

Causes of syncope

1 Reflex (neutrally mediated) syncope
   - ➤ vasovagal syncope (simple faint)
   - ➤ breath-holding attacks
   - ➤ reflex anoxic seizure
   - ➤ postural hypotension.
2 Syncope of cardiac origin
   - ➤ Cardiac arrhythmia:
     - ➤ complete heart block
     - ➤ long QTc syndrome (causing polymorphic ventricular tachycardia)
     - ➤ ventricular tachycardia (often monomorphic)
     - ➤ sick sinus syndrome and SA node dysfunction
   - ➤ Structural/functional heart defects:
     - ➤ aortic stenosis
     - ➤ hypertrophic cardiomyopathy
     - ➤ restrictive cardiomyopathy
   - ➤ Pulmonary hypertension.
3 Non-cardiac in origin
   - ➤ benign paroxysmal vertigo
   - ➤ migraine
   - ➤ fabricated or induced illness.

Clinical features

- ❯ Pale
- ❯ Hypotensive
- ❯ Sweaty
- ❯ Tachycardic/bradycardic
- ❯ Palpitations
- ❯ Seizure (secondary to hypoxia)

Investigations

- ❯ ECG
- ❯ 24-hour ECG recording/Cardiomemo
- ❯ Echo
- ❯ BP (lying and standing)
- ❯ Blood sugar
- ❯ Tilt Test

SYNDROMES ASSOCIATED WITH CARDIAC ABNORMALITIES

Syndrome	Genetics	Cardiac features	Other features
Alagille syndrome	Autosomal dominant with variable expression. Mutations in JAG-1 and NOTCH 2	Peripheral pulmonary stenosis	• Hypoplasia of intralobular bile ducts • Characteristic facies with thin triangular face, prominent forehead and deep set eyes • Vertebral arch abnormalities, butterfly vertebrae • Renal tract anomalies • Associated mental retardation
CHARGE association	Sporadic inheritance	PDA ASD/VSD/AVSD Tetralogy of Fallot Double outlet right ventricle Aortic arch abnormalities	**C:** Coloboma **H:** Heart defect **A:** choanal Atresia **R:** Retarded growth and development **G:** Genital hypoplasia **E:** Ear anomalies
DiGeorge syndrome	Microdeletion on chromosome 22 Sporadic inheritance	Interrupted aortic arch Conotruncal defect Truncus arteriosus Tetralogy of Fallot Familial VSD	• 22q11.2 deletion • Abnormal development of fourth branchial arch and third/fourth pharyngeal pouches • Cleft palate • Absent thymus with T-cell deficiency • Hypoparathyroidism and hypocalcaemia
Down syndrome	Trisomy 21 (95%) Translocation (4%) Mosaic (1%)	AVSD/VSD ASD PDA	• Characteristic facies with almond-shaped eyes, epicanthic folds, up-slanting palpebral fissures and protruding tongue • Single palmar crease • Increased risk of leukaemia • Associated with hypothyroidism, dementia, duodenal atresia and atlantoaxial instability • Increasing risk with increased maternal age

(continued)

Syndrome	Genetics	Cardiac features	Other features
Edwards syndrome	Trisomy 18	VSD/ASD PDA Coarctation of the aorta Bicuspid aortic valve	• Characteristic facies with cleft lip/palate, micrognathia, low set ears and microcephaly • Overlapping fingers • Rocker-bottom feet • Renal anomalies • Very poor prognosis with 90% dead in first year
Ehlers–Danlos syndrome	Autosomal dominant Occasionally autosomal recessive	Aortic dissection Aortic regurgitation	• Defective type 3 collagen (nine different types have been described) • Marked skin hyperelasticity • Poor wound healing • Hyperextensible joints • Risk of joint dislocation • Easy bruising • Associated with varicose veins, congenital diaphragmatic hernia and hiatus hernia
Goldenhar syndrome (oculo-auriculo-vertebral dysplasia)	Sporadic inheritance	VSD Tetralogy of Fallot	• Abnormal development of first and second branchial arches • Facial asymmetry: hemifacial hyposomia • Right side of face more severely affected • Cleft lip and palate • Coloboma of the eyelid • Conductive or sensorineural deafness • Malformed pinna • Renal abnormalities • Vertebral anomalies
Holt–Oram syndrome	Autosomal dominant with variable expression	ASD VSD	• Limb defects: radial/ulna hypoplasia • Hypoplastic thumbs • Limb reduction defects • Absent pectoralis major • Vertebral anomalies
Jervell and Lange–Nielsen syndrome	Autosomal recessive inheritance	Prolonged QT interval Ventricular tachycardia	• Sensorineural deafness

Syndrome	Genetics	Cardiac features	Other features
Klippel-Feil sequence	Sporadic inheritance Female : male = 2 : 1	VSD	• Short webbed neck • Low posterior hairline • Congenital fusion of the cervical vertebrae into a single bony mass • Kyphoscoliosis • Ocular defects: nystagmus, squints • Cleft palate • Occipitocervical instability • Syringomyelia and syringobulbia • Associated deafness
Leopard syndrome	Mode of inheritance not fully understood	ECG abnormalities (left axis deviation, long PR interval, right bundle branch block) Risk of arrhythmias high	**L:** Lentigines **E:** ECG abnormalities **O:** Ocular hypertelorism **P:** Pulmonary stenosis **A:** Abnormalities of the genitalia **R:** Retarded growth **D:** Deafness
Marfan syndrome	Autosomal dominant with variable expression Due to a mutation of the fibrillin gene on chromosome 15	Mitral valve prolapsed Aortic regurgitation Aortic dissection	• Tall with long limbs, arm span greater than height • Arachnodactyly • Pectus excavatum or pectum carinatum • Kyphoscoliosis • High arched palate • Ectopia lentis, with lens dislocation up and outwards (cc to homocystinuria) • Increased joint laxity • Increased risk of pneumothorax
Noonan syndrome	Autosomal dominant with variable transmission Chromosome 12	Pulmonary stenosis ASD Cardiomyopathy Septal hypertrophy	• Normal karyotype • Look phenotypically similar to children with Turner syndrome • Triangular facies • Short stature • Feeding difficulties common in the neonatal period • Mild mental retardation • Vertebral defects • Cryptoorchidism

(*continued*)

Syndrome	Genetics	Cardiac features	Other features
Patau syndrome	Trisomy 13 or 15	VSD/ASD PDA Coarctation of the aorta Bicuspid aortic valve	• Renal anomalies • Midline facial cleft • Holoprosencephaly
Romano–Ward syndrome	Autosomal dominant	Prolonged QT interval Ventricular tachycardia	• Family history of recurrent syncope or sudden death
Treacher–Collins syndrome	Autosomal dominant with variable expression 50% new mutation rate	VSD	• A first branchial arch defect • Characteristic facies with external ear canal defects, cleft palate, mandibular hypoplasia, absence of lower lid eyelashes and down-slanting palpebral fissures • Usually of normal intelligence • Conductive and sensorineural deafness
Tuberous sclerosis	Autosomal dominant with 70% new mutation rate Chromosome 9 Gene located 9q34	Rhabdomyomas	• Shagreen patch • Amelanotic naevi (ash-leaf patch) • Adenoma sebaceum • Subungual fibroma • Cafe au lait patches • Developmental delay • Epilepsy • Renal anomalies • Intracranial calcification • Gliotic hamartomas may undergo malignant change
Turner syndrome	45XO Mosaics also occur	Coarctation of the aorta Bicuspid aortic valve	• Short stature • Cubitus valgus • Webbed neck • Widely spaced nipples • Renal anomalies: horseshoe kidney • Ovarian dysgenesis • Lower than average IQ

Syndrome	Genetics	Cardiac features	Other features
VACTERL association	Sporadic inheritance	Tetralogy of Fallot VSD	**V:** Vertebral anomalies, hemi or bifid vertebrae **A:** Anorectal malformations **C:** Cardiac defects **T:** Tracheo-oesophageal fistula **E:** Oesophageal atresia **R:** Renal defects: VUR, renal dysplasia **L:** Limb abnormalities, radial dysplasia
Williams syndrome	Sporadic inheritance Microdeletion on Chromosome 7	Supravalvular aortic stenosis Branch pulmonary artery stenosis	• Characteristic facies with elfin-like features, small mandible, depressed nasal bridge, long smooth philtrum and prominent cheeks • Enamel hypoplasia • Mild–moderate mental retardation • Friendly personality: 'cocktail party chatter' • Renal artery stenosis and hypertension

Tetralogy of Fallot
Total anomalous pulmonary venous drainage (TAPVD)
Transplant cardiology
Transposition of the great arteries (TGA)
Treacher–Collins syndrome – *see* Syndromes associated with cardiac
    abnormalities
Tricuspid atresia
Truncus arteriosus
Tuberous sclerosis – *see* Syndromes associated with cardiac
    abnormalities
Turner syndrome – *see* Syndromes associated with cardiac
    abnormalities

TETRALOGY OF FALLOT

➤ Accounts for approximately 6% of all congenital heart lesions.
➤ The most common cause of cyanotic congenital heart disease.
➤ Decreased pulmonary blood flow with a right–left shunt.
➤ Consists of four cardinal features:
  1 Right ventricular outflow tract obstruction (pulmonary stenosis)
  2 Ventricular septal defect – perimembranous
  3 Overriding of the aorta
  4 Right ventricular hypertrophy.

Figure 6.56 shows the anatomical defects.

Pathophysiology

The VSD is usually large and non-restrictive, which allows equalisation of pressure between the right and left ventricles.

As the right ventricle contracts in the presence of marked pulmonary stenosis, blood is shunted across the VSD into the aorta, resulting in *cyanosis*.

The pulmonary stenosis can affect both the infundibulum and the pulmonary valve.

If the pulmonary blood flow is severely restricted by the obstruction to the right ventricular outflow, the circulation may be supplemented by collateral vessels.

The degree of right to left shunting through the VSD is determined by the severity of the obstruction of the right ventricular outflow tract; this in turn determines the severity of cyanosis.

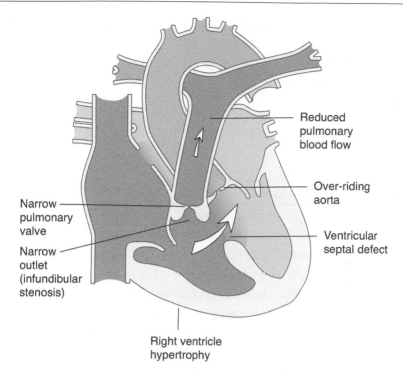

FIGURE 6.56 The anatomy of tetralogy of Fallot

If the pulmonary valve stenosis is mild there will be equal left to right shunting across the VSD, and the child may then be 'pink' (acyanotic).

Right ventricular hypertrophy develops secondary to increased right ventricular pressure.

Clinical course

Cyanosis may not be present at birth.

As the child grows, cyanosis becomes more pronounced as a result of increasing infundibular hypertrophy with subsequent obstruction.

'**Hypoxic spells**' are often associated with feeding, crying, exertion and irritability. The baby becomes increasingly cyanosed and restless. There is a reduction of an already compromised pulmonary blood flow. The intensity of the murmur decreases during an attack. The exact underlying aetiology is poorly understood but probably due to spasm of the infundibular muscle which causes the decrease in pulmonary blood flow.

Prolonged attacks can lead to:

➤ hypoxia
➤ metabolic acidosis
➤ convulsions
➤ myocardial infarction
➤ cerebrovascular accidents.

They can be life threatening, but if managed promptly are rarely fatal. Management:

➤ knee-chest position

➤ supplemental high-flow oxygen

➤ morphine

➤ consideration of bicarbonate

➤ β-blockers are used to prevent spells.

Cardiac investigations

Investigation	Main features
ECG	Right ventricular hypertrophy
	Right axis deviation
	Upright T wave in V1
	Tall P wave, sometimes bifid
Chest X-ray	Decreased pulmonary vascular markings
	Cardiothoracic ratio usually within normal limits
	Right-sided aortic arch in approximately 20% of cases
Echocardiography	Demonstrates the four cardinal anatomical features:
	1 Right ventricular outflow tract obstruction
	2 VSD
	3 Overriding of the aorta
	4 Right ventricular hypertrophy
Cardiac catheterisation	Useful to define the anatomy of collateral vessels
	Mean arterial pressure is usually normal
	Systolic pressure in the right ventricle can equal systemic pressure

Complications:

➤ myocardial infarction

➤ cerebrovascular accident

➤ cerebral thromboses

➤ cerebral ischaemia

➤ congestive heart failure

➤ infective endocarditis

➤ brain abscess.

Palliative surgical intervention

Babies presenting in the early neonatal period with severe cyanosis have a significant obstruction of the right ventricular outflow tract. A systemic to pulmonary artery shunt increases pulmonary artery blood flow.

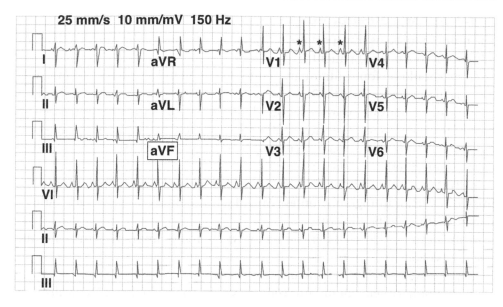

FIGURE 6.57 Electrocardiogram from an infant with tetralogy of Fallot. The ECG in tetralogy of Fallot shows prominent P waves in V1(*) suggesting right atrial enlargement. There are also prominent right ventricular forces (tall R waves in V1), an upright T wave in V1, and a marked rightward axis (rS in I and aVL and qR in aVR) suggesting right ventricular hypertrophy.

Blalock–Taussig shunt: a modified procedure uses an artificial conduit from the subclavian to pulmonary artery (*see* page 82).

Corrective surgical intervention: total corrective repair is usually performed electively at around 6 months of age. It involves:
➤ closure of the VSD
➤ enlargement of the right ventricular outflow tract.

The surgical risk is approximately 2%–5%.

Clinical features
❯ Cyanosis
❯ Short stature
❯ Loud ejection systolic murmur
❯ +/– systolic thrill
❯ Single second heart sounds
❯ Dyspnoea
❯ Finger clubbing
❯ +/– developmental delay

Investigations
❯ ECG
❯ CXR
❯ Echo
❯ Cardiac catheterisation

TOTAL ANOMALOUS PULMONARY VENOUS DRAINAGE (TAPVD)

The pulmonary veins transport the oxygenated blood from the lungs back to the left atrium in a normal patient.

There should be four pulmonary veins (two right and two left). Normal anatomy is discussed in Chapter 2.

Total anomalous pulmonary venous drainage describes the situation when all four of the pulmonary veins do not drain into the left atria; they return direct to the systemic venous circulation (therefore do not deliver oxygenated blood to the systemic arterial circulation).

TAPVD is an example of cyanotic heart disease and has the potential to be missed on echocardiography unless careful effort is made to view each pulmonary vein; this can be difficult.

TAPVD can be classified depending on where the pulmonary veins enter the systemic venous circulation.

➤ Supra-cardiac TAPVD (Figure 6.58A):
  ➤ pulmonary veins drain into venous system above the heart (typically the innominate vein or SVC)
  ➤ most common type of TAPVD.

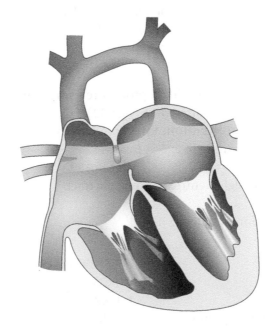

FIGURE 6.58A Supracardiac TAPVD (pulmonary veins draining to the innominate vein)

➤ Cardiac TAPVD (Figure 6.58B):
  ➤ pulmonary veins drain into the right side of the heart (typically the coronary sinus)
  ➤ second most common type of TAPVD.

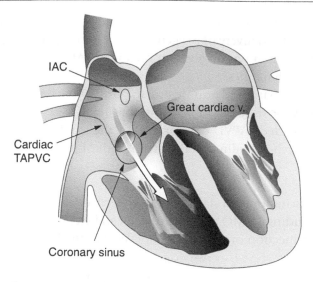

FIGURE 6.58B Cardiac TAPVD (pulmonary veins draining to the right atria via the coronary sinus)

➤ Infra-cardiac TAPVD (Figure 6.58C):
  ➤ pulmonary veins drain into the venous system below the diaphragm (typically the portal venous system or IVC)
  ➤ although least common, can be the most serious as the pulmonary venous system is more likely to be obstructed than the above examples.

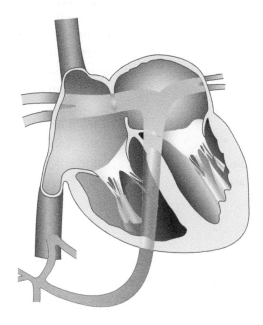

FIGURE 6.58C Infracardiac TAPVD (pulmonary veins draining to the portal venous system)

In TAPVD (as with many cyanotic heart lesions) there needs to be mixing at the foramen ovale for delivery of oxygenated blood to the systemic arterial circulation. The PDA is often not involved in mixing in TAPVD. Prostin may actually worsen the haemodynamics!

If there is good mixing and non-obstructed TAPVD the baby can be quite well, with only mild cyanosis (saturations around 90%).

If there is obstructed TAPVD or poor mixing, the child can be very unwell and progress rapidly to heart failure in the first month of life.

Management
➤ Suitable resuscitation and stabilisation as needed (may need significant support, including ECMO as if obstructed can be critically unwell).
➤ Surgical reconnection of the pulmonary veins to the left atrium.

Clinical features

Non-obstructed TAPVD
> Similar to large ASD
> Failure to thrive
> Short of breath
> Recurrent lower respiratory tract infections
> May or may not have cyanosis (mild)
> RV heave
> Split second heart sound
> Pulmonary flow murmur

Obstructed TAPVD
> Cyanosis (severe)
> Tachypnoea/tachycardia
> Respiratory distress
> Cardiogenic shock
> Features of heart failure
> Loud second heart sound
> Often no murmur
> Hepatomegaly

Investigations

1 CXR can be normal. It may show a 'snowman in a storm' appearance. This is a 'figure 8 shape' of the heart with increased pulmonary vascular markings.
2 ECG may demonstrate a sinus tachycardia with evidence of RV hypertrophy.
3 Echo will demonstrate the anatomy of the pulmonary veins and cardiac function. It may show dilated portal veins if infracardiac TAPVD.
4 Further imaging may be needed to demarcate the pulmonary veins if unable to clearly assess on echo. MRI or diagnostic cardiac catheterisation would be good for this.

Partial anomalous pulmonary venous drainage (PAPVD)
This congenital heart disease describes the situation when at least one pulmonary vein connects correctly to the left atria but one to three of the pulmonary veins drain elsewhere into the systemic venous circulation (Figure 6.59).

The site of drainage can be varied. It can be a difficult diagnosis to make unless all four pulmonary veins are assessed carefully on echocardiography.

Associated with Noonan and Turner syndromes.

Often found with sinus venosus atrial septal defects (*see* page 75).

Presentation and course is often much less severe than TAPVD.

Management is similar to TAPVD.

TRANSPLANT CARDIOLOGY

Cardiac transplantation has been used in children for over 20 years; the first attempt at a cardiac transplant in a child was performed in 1968. This was unsuccessful.

Since that time major improvements have occurred in paediatric heart transplantation and 2011 data from the International Society of Heart & Lung Transplantation (ISHLT) suggests:

➤ over 70% average survival at 5 years

➤ 50% average survival at 15 years.

Indications for paediatric heart transplant include:

➤ cardiomyopathy (any type)

➤ complex congenital heart disease

➤ retransplantation due to heart failure or rejection of the previous heart.

The commonest indication for paediatric heart transplant in the UK is cardiomyopathy.

Around 400 paediatric heart transplants are performed worldwide each year.

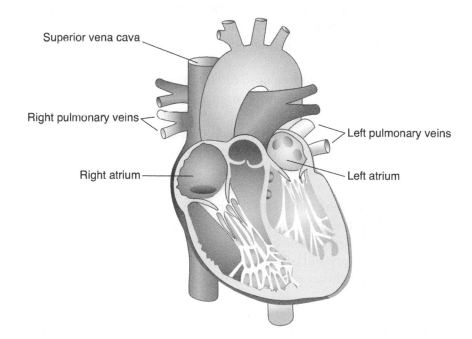

Superior vena cava

Right pulmonary veins

Left pulmonary veins

Right atrium

Left atrium

FIGURE 6.59 PAPVD

The average wait time for a donor heart depends upon many factors, including the following.
➤ Age and size of child, severity of illness, other children on the waiting list.
➤ Generally, infants wait longer than older children.
➤ The average wait time in the UK for a donor heart in paediatrics is 93 days.

Prior to transplantation children may need a variety of management methods:
➤ heart failure medications (e.g. diuretics, ACE inhibitors, β-blockers)
➤ inotropic support (e.g. dobutamine)
➤ palliative surgical procedures
➤ 'bridge to transplant' mechanical support (e.g. ECMO, Berlin Heart)
➤ ventilation.

Complications post paediatric heart transplant include:
➤ rejection of the organ (see below)
➤ hypertension
➤ pericardial effusion
➤ accelerated coronary artery disease
➤ complications of the immunosuppression
  ➤ infection risk
  ➤ impaired renal function
  ➤ bone marrow suppression
  ➤ malignancy
  ➤ specific side-effects exist for each immunosuppressant: cyclosporin →
    hirsutism; tacrolimus → alopecia; steroids → Cushingoid appearance,
    growth cessation, weight gain.

Following transplantation children need careful management to observe for signs of rejection (often non-specific) and to manage any of the complications mentioned above.
  The transplanted heart has no autonomic supply and is denervated. This means ischaemic events will be pain free (and may present with sudden cardiac death). It also means that β-blockers have no effect.
  Long-term follow-up:
➤ usually managed by the transplant centre with additional support from the patient's local cardiac unit (each unit will have varying policies)
➤ frequent blood investigations to monitor FBC, U&E.
➤ regular cardiac biopsy and coronary angiography
➤ regular ECGs and echo assessment.

Cardiac rejection is a significant complication of heart transplantation.
➤ Often presents in a very non-specific way, and should always be kept in a differential diagnosis of a child with a known heart transplant.

➤ Can present acutely or with a more chronic course.

Clinical features of rejection include:
➤ pyrexia (may be low grade)
➤ lethargy and fatigue
➤ weight gain (a sign of fluid retention)
➤ evidence of heart failure:
　➢ tachycardia (often when at rest and persistent)
　➢ gallop rhythm (third heart sound)
　➢ hypotension/poor peripheral perfusion
　➢ pleural effusions.

Investigations when rejection is suspected include the following.
➤ Echo:
　➢ will show reduced cardiac function (diastolic dysfunction first)
　➢ mitral regurgitation
　➢ pericardial effusions.
➤ ECG:
　➢ sinus tachycardia
　➢ may demonstrate ventricular ectopic beats
　➢ low-voltage QRS complexes.
➤ CXR:
　➢ cardiomegaly
　➢ pleural effusions
　➢ pulmonary oedema
➤ Cardiac biopsy.

Rejection is treated with methylprednisolone with alteration in immunosuppressants and any additional support as needed. Retransplantation may be required in some cases.

When dealing with a child with a transplanted heart *always* discuss the case with the transplant centre as these children often need a multidisciplinary approach to problems (transplant physician, cardiologist, immunologist, general paediatrician, specialist nurses, and psychologists).

TRANSPOSITION OF THE GREAT ARTERIES (TGA)
Transposition of the great arteries is a cyanotic congenital cardiac lesion.

It accounts for approximately 5%–6% of cases of all congenital heart lesions.

It is the second commonest cause of cyanotic heart disease, but is the most common cyanotic heart defect detected in the neonatal period (tetralogy of Fallot is the commonest overall cyanotic defect, but often not diagnosed until infancy).

There is a male predominance with a 3 : 1 male to female ratio.

Anatomy

The aorta is connected to the right ventricle and the pulmonary artery to the left ventricle (*see* Figure 6.60).

This is sometimes described as concordant atrioventricular and discordant ventriculoarterial connections.

There are two parallel circulations:

➤ **systemic venous return:** blood passes from the right atrium to the right ventricle and into the aorta

➤ **pulmonary venous return:** blood returns to the left atrium to the left ventricle and back into the pulmonary arteries.

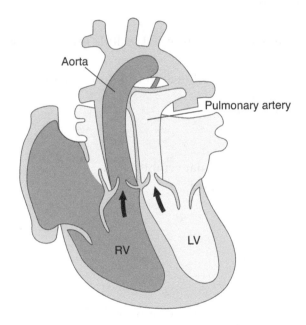

FIGURE 6.60 Complete transposition of the great arteries

It is essential for survival that there is an associated defect that allows mixing of the blood.

Common shunts that are present include:

➤ VSD

➤ ASD or PFO

➤ PDA.

Since the systemic and pulmonary circulations are in parallel rather than in series the presence of an associated defect allows mixing of blood between the two circulations.

TGA is often complicated by other lesions; e.g. VSD, pulmonary stenosis or coarctation of the aorta.

Pathophysiology

There is a loss of the normal sequential relationship between the systemic and pulmonary circulations.

As the pulmonary vascular resistance decreases there is an increase in pulmonary blood flow and correspondingly the left side of the heart becomes volume overloaded.

Heart failure may occur as a consequence of:

➤ low arterial PO_2
➤ progressive metabolic acidosis
➤ myocardial depression
➤ volume overload of the left side of the heart.

As in all cyanotic congenital heart defects the severity of the hypoxia will depend upon:

1 The adequacy of mixing between the two parallel circuits through the shunt
2 The volume of pulmonary blood flow.

Clinical presentation

Most babies with TGA will present with cyanosis within the first week of life.

Those with a small ASD or patent foramen ovale will present earlier compared to babies with a large VSD, due to more severe cyanosis.

On auscultation the second heart sound may be single and accentuated.

There may be a systolic murmur if a VSD is present which increases in intensity as the pulmonary vascular resistance falls.

These babies remain hypoxic, and performing a hyperoxic test demonstrates hypoxaemia unresponsive to oxygen therapy.

Investigations

Investigation	Findings
ECG	Right ventricular hypertrophy
	+/– left ventricular hypertrophy = biventricular hypertrophy
CXR	Increased cardiothoracic ratio
	Increased pulmonary vascular markings
	Narrow cardiac pedicle
	Cardiac contour has an 'egg-on-side' appearance
ABG	Low PaO_2 (with failure to increase with hyperoxia (nitrogen washout)
	Progressive metabolic acidosis due to low cardiac output
Echo	Demonstrates the origin of the pulmonary artery from the left ventricle and the aorta from the right ventricle
	Plus any associated cardiac defects

Management

Supportive care with respiratory and cardiovascular function.

Avoid oxygen; accept saturations in the 70% range.

Commence prostaglandin therapy (*see* page 34) to keep PDA open.

Arrange urgent transfer to paediatric cardiology unit for:

➤ **balloon atrial septostomy** (*see* Rashkind procedure, page 171)

➤ Corrective surgical repair:

➣ *arterial switch procedure:* anatomical correction is achieved as the pulmonary artery and the aorta are transacted and switched over, including the repositioning of the coronary arteries. This is now gold standard (*see* page 171)

➣ *Mustard or Senning operation:* a baffle diverts the systemic venous return at atrial level (*see* page 142)

➣ *Rastelli procedure:* redirection of blood flow at ventricular level (*see* page 171)

Clinical features

❯ Routine finding of cyanosis on newborn check

❯ May have no signs on examination other than low saturations

❯ Cyanosis

❯ Split or single second heart sound

❯ +/– systolic murmur

❯ Tachypnoea and tachycardia

Investigations

❯ ECG

❯ CXR

❯ Echo

❯ ABG + nitrogen washout

TRICUSPID ATRESIA

Describes the failure of a tricuspid valve to develop, resulting in a hypoplastic right heart type syndrome.

It is the third most common cyanotic heart disease, after tetralogy of Fallot and transposition of the great arteries (TGA).

Tricuspid atresia is often associated with other cardiac defects (including VSD and TGA).

Higher incidence in maternal diabetes mellitus.

The anatomy of tricuspid atresia is shown in Figure 6.61.

In tricuspid atresia blood cannot pass from the RA to the RV:

➤ blood shunts right to left through the foreman ovale and a ductus arteriosus

➤ the blood flow to the RV and then onto the lungs is usually via a ventricular septal defect

➤ as a result there is mixing of blood so these children are cyanotic.

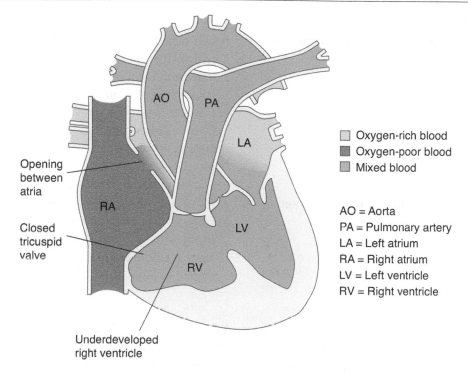

Oxygen-rich blood
Oxygen-poor blood
Mixed blood

AO = Aorta
PA = Pulmonary artery
LA = Left atrium
RA = Right atrium
LV = Left ventricle
RV = Right ventricle

FIGURE 6.61 Tricuspid atresia

These children may be diagnosed in the antenatal period on anomaly screening. If not, they usually present with significant cyanosis soon after birth, depending on the degree of intra-atrial shunting.

Management in the initial period will depend on the degree of pulmonary blood flow.

➤ If low pulmonary blood flow:
  ➢ will be severely hypoxic and will need prostaglandin to maintain duct patency
  ➢ an emergency BT shunt may be needed.

If pulmonary blood flow is very high (often seen with large VSD)
➤ a PA band may be needed
➤ diuretics may be needed.

In all cases palliative surgery will be required.
➤ Usually, the staged Fontan procedure is used, to produce a single ventricle system.
  ➢ *See* Norwood procedure, page 146 and Fontan circulation, page 111.

Clinical features

> Antenatal diagnosis on fetal echo

If low pulmonary blood flow:
> Cyanosis
> Murmur of VSD
> Cardiogenic shock

If high pulmonary blood flow:
> Less cyanosis
> Present with cardiac failure and volume overload

Investigations

1 ECG usually shows a sinus rhythm with a superior QRS axis. There may be evidence of right atrial enlargement (P-pulmonale).
2 CXR can demonstrate cardiomegaly (due to enlargement of the right atria as no blood can exit into the right ventricle). Pulmonary vascular markings are usually reduced due to lower pulmonary blood flow.
3 Echo will demonstrate the anatomy of the tricuspid atresia, along with associated defects and help assess degree of pulmonary blood flow.

TRUNCUS ARTERIOSUS

Truncus arteriosus is a congenital heart defect where there is a single (truncal) vessel leaving the ventricle with a single (truncal) valve.
➤ This single vessel gives rise to the aorta, pulmonary artery and coronary arteries.

The anatomy of truncus arteriosus can vary depending on how the pulmonary arteries appear. A classification system exists, but is not relevant for this book. Figure 6.62 shows one example of truncus arteriosus.

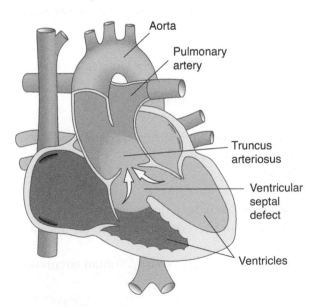

FIGURE 6.62 Truncus arteriosus

The incidence is ~10 per 100 000 live births.

Truncus arteriosus is associated with:
➤ DiGeorge syndrome (22q11 microdeletion)
➤ velocardiofacial syndrome
➤ maternal diabetes mellitus.

Truncus arteriosus is frequently associated with other cardiac defects:
➤ dysplastic truncal valve
➤ interrupted aortic arch
➤ coronary artery anomalies
➤ ventricular septal defects
➤ atrial septal defects
➤ many other defects can be present; careful assessment is needed.

The infant with truncus arteriosus can have a varied presentation, depending on the degree of pulmonary blood flow:
➤ typically present with a heart failure presentation due to high pulmonary blood flow
➤ may present with only mild cyanosis (saturations around 90%)
➤ can present with features of other defects (e.g. interrupted aortic arch)
   ➢ cardiogenic shock (*see* page 217)

Management will involve the following.
➤ Initial stabilisation as per APLS/NLS guidelines.
➤ Often need diuretics to manage heart failure pre surgery.
➤ May need prostaglandin for treatment of aortic arch defects, but do not need prostaglandin for the truncus arteriosus itself; it is not a duct-dependent circulation.
➤ Surgical correction is often indicated as soon as symptoms appear.
➤ Correction of the associated defect may be needed.

Clinical features
❭ Antenatal diagnosis
❭ Cyanosis (mild)
❭ Heart failure symptoms (poor feeding, sweating, respiratory distress, tachycardia, tachypnoea)
❭ Murmur of truncal valve stenosis/regurgitation may be present or VSD
❭ Cardiogenic shock if associated duct-dependent lesion present

Investigations
1 CXR may show cardiomegaly and increased pulmonary vascular markings.
2 ECG is often normal. May demonstrate biventricular hypertrophy.
3 Echo will give the diagnosis and reveal the anatomy of the truncus and associated defects.

(*continued*)

Clinical features

> Maybe dysmorphic (associated with syndromes)

Investigations

4 Diagnostic catheterisation may be needed to delineate complex vasculature anatomy.

5 FISH for 22q11 microdeletion (as high association with DiGeorge syndrome).

VACTERL association – *see* Syndromes associated with cardiac
abnormalities
Ventricular septal defect (VSD)
Ventricular tachycardia (VT)

VENTRICULAR SEPTAL DEFECT (VSD)

The ventricular septum divides the left and right ventricles. Any communication through this septum is known as a ventricular septal defect.

VSD is the commonest congenital heart defect, accounting for 30% of all the congenital heart defects.

The incidence of VSD is quoted as around 5500 per 100 000 live births.
➤ It may be higher than this.
➤ Many VSDs are insignificant and so may never be discovered.
➤ VSDs often spontaneously close – sometimes before a diagnosis is made.

VSD is often an isolated defect, but can form part of other lesions including:
➤ tetralogy of Fallot
➤ pulmonary atresia with VSD
➤ transposition of the great arteries.

Associations with a VSD include:
➤ Down syndrome
➤ Patau syndrome (trisomy 13)
➤ Edwards syndrome (trisomy 18)
➤ Holt–Oram syndrome.

The majority of VSDs are haemodynamically insignificant and are detected by the incidental finding of a murmur during auscultation of the chest for some other reasons.

The majority of small and moderate VSDs are often not seen in the antenatal period. Large VSDs and VSDs with other conditions may be identified antenatally.

Moderate to large VSDs may have haemodynamic consequences and present with infant heart failure.
➤ Significant left to right shunting.
  ➤ This causes high pulmonary blood flow and volume overloading of the LA and LV (due to high pulmonary venous return to the left side of the heart).

➤ This can cause a reduction in systemic cardiac output and high pulmonary pressures; it results in heart failure.

➤ The significant left to right shunt is due to the formation of a large hole with lower RV pressures than LV pressures (high gradient). This is made worse as the neonate grows; the pulmonary vascular resistance falls and so does the RV pressure. The left to right shunting therefore increases.

➤ High pulmonary vascular resistance in the neonatal period acts as a protective mechanism.

➤ As a result, the infant often presents in heart failure when the pulmonary vascular resistance falls.

➤ Damage to pulmonary vascular bed.

➤ This occurs because of the high pulmonary blood flow.

➤ Over time this damage can become irreversible and cause pulmonary hypertension.

➤ This can lead to Eisenmenger syndrome in later life (*see* page 106).

VSD can be called small, moderate or large in size.

➤ A small hole → restriction in flow → higher velocity blood through the VSD → Louder murmur → +/– thrill.

➤ A large hole → no restriction in flow → low-velocity, high-volume blood through the VSD → quiet murmur with no thrill +/– heave.

VSDs are then often classified on their anatomical location.

1 Muscular VSD (Figure 6.63A):
➤ the VSD occurs in the muscular proportion of the septum (i.e. mid to lower septum)
➤ all the edges of the VSD are made up of ventricular muscle
➤ can have single or multiple defects ('Swiss Cheese Defect')
➤ small muscular VSDs likely to close spontaneously.

2 Perimembranous VSD:
➤ the VSD occurs in the membranous portion of the septum (i.e. the upper septum)
➤ this defect has close proximity to the inlet (mitral and tricuspid) and outlet (aortic and pulmonary) valves
➤ can still spontaneously close, but less likely to do so than the muscular VSDs
➤ Figure 6.63B demonstrates a perimembranous VSD high up in the septum.

The majority of VSDs do not give any long-term problems. However, follow-up is needed to ensure that:
➤ as the pulmonary vascular resistance falls the hole does not allow high left to right shunt

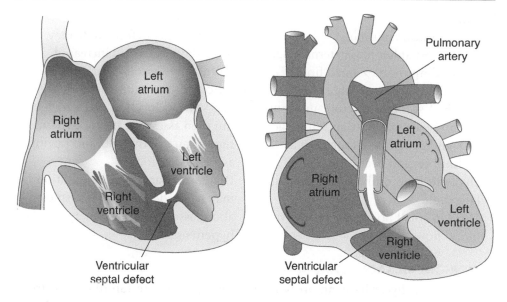

FIGURE 6.63A Muscular VSD

FIGURE 6.63B Perimembranous VSD

> the cardiac function remains good
> there is no evidence of raised pulmonary artery pressures
> there is no secondary damage to the valves of the heart, due to the flow through the VSD.

Management includes the following.
> Follow-up for small holes.
> Medical management of heart failure (e.g. diuretics, ACE inhibitors).
> PA band to reduced pulmonary blood flow (often only done in small neonates less than 3 kg to give them time to grow).
> Surgical closure of the VSD.
> Cardiac catheter device closure of muscular VSD is undertaken at some centres, in a similar way to ASD device closures.

Clinical features
> Antenatal diagnosis (large defects)
> Asymptomatic
> Incidental murmur detected
> Recurrent lower respiratory tract infections
> Signs and symptoms of heart failure (moderate–large defects) – *see* page 84

Investigations
1 ECG will be normal in small VSDs. In larger defects it may show sinus tachycardia, LV hypertrophy and in some cases biventricular hypertrophy.

(continued)

> Murmur
> ✓ Pansystolic murmur
> ✓ Loudest at left lower sternal edge
> ✓ Loud murmur → small hole
> ✓ Quiet murmur → large hole
> ✓ NB: A soft mid-diastolic murmur can be heard at the apex in large, significant VSDs along with a loud second heart sound
> Dynamic praecordium with heave in large hole
> Thrill in small holes with restrictive blood flow

2 CXR will be normal in small VSD. In larger defects there may be cardiomegaly and increased pulmonary vascular markings.
3 Echo will determine the presence of a VSD, its location and size. It can then assess the haemodynamic significance of the VSD and identify associated lesions.
4 Diagnostic cardiac catheterisation may be needed if there is suspicion about associated pulmonary hypertension.

VENTRICULAR TACHYCARDIA (VT)

Ventricular tachycardia is an arrhythmia many people are familiar with from resuscitation training. However, VT is not always a cardiac arrest rhythm.

VT is defined as:
➤ three or more consecutive beats
➤ arising from the ventricles
➤ at a rate greater than 120 beats per minute.

ECG features of VT therefore include:
➤ a wide complex QRS
➤ regular QRS
➤ QRS usually all the same shape and size (monomorphic VT) – polymorphic VT is when the QRS amplitude and axis varies; associated with long QT
➤ tachycardia.

This is shown in the rhythm strip in Figure 6.64.

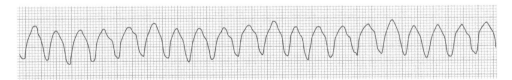

FIGURE 6.64 Ventricular tachycardia

Sustained VT is when this arrhythmia lasts for more than 30 seconds. Non-sustained VT is when the arrhythmia lasts for less than 30 seconds.

Causes of VT include the following.

➤ Idiopathic
➤ Metabolic disturbances:
  ➢ hypoxia
  ➢ electrolyte disturbances: hyperkalaemia, hypokalaemia, hypomagnesaemia and hypocalcaemia
  ➢ acidosis
  ➢ hypoglycaemia
➤ Inherited disorders:
  ➢ long QT syndrome
  ➢ Brugada syndrome
➤ Inflammatory heart disease:
  ➢ myocarditis
➤ Structural heart disease:
  ➢ cardiomyopathy
  ➢ tetralogy of Fallot
  ➢ coronary artery abnormalities
➤ Toxins:
  ➢ drug overdose, e.g. digoxin, tricyclic antidepressants, salicylates
  ➢ inotropes
➤ Trauma:
  ➢ cardiac surgery
  ➢ chest trauma
  ➢ direct ventricular stimulation (e.g. central lines into ventricle)

Children with VT can have situations where they have an inadequate cardiac output to generate a pulse (so called 'pulseless' VT). This is actually quite rare.

The majority of children with VT will present as with any other arrhythmia (e.g. palpitations). See clinical features below.

Management of the VT will depend on the clinical state of the child. VT has the potential to rapidly deteriorate into ventricular fibrillation (VF).

In an acute presentation management will depend on the degree of haemo-dynamic compromise present (for algorithm *see Advanced Paediatric Life Support: The Practical Approach (APLS)*, 5th Edition (Wiley-Blackwell; 2011)).

➤ Haemodynamic compromise:
  ➢ rapid DC cardioversion is indicated (1 J/kg for first shock then 2 J/kg): if with pulse – synchronised (plus sedation); if pulseless – managed as a cardiac arrest with asynchronous shock (for algorithm *see Advanced Paediatric Life Support: The Practical Approach (APLS)*, 5th Edition (Wiley-Blackwell; 2011))
  ➢ correct underlying cause.

➤ No haemodynamic compromise:
  ➢ correct underlying cause
  ➢ seek paediatric cardiology advice as soon as possible: consider DC cardioversion; may respond to IV amiodarone or lidocaine infusion.
➤ The long-term management is very specific to the underlying cause. This can range from medication (e.g. β-blockers in long QT), to radiofrequency ablation to insertion of implantable cardioverter defibrillators (ICDs).

Clinical features

> Asymptomatic, found by chance on ECG
> Palpitations
> Syncope
> Heart failure
> Features of underlying cause
> Tachycardia
> Haemodynamic compromise (low BP, poor perfusion, reduced consciousness)
> Cardiac arrest

Investigations

1 ECG (Figure 6.64) demonstrates a regular wide complex QRS with rapid rate. When cardioverted it may show a reason for the VT (e.g. long QT, evidence of hyperkalaemia).
2 Echo can show structure and function of heart.
3 U&E/LFT/Bone Profile to assess for underlying cause.
4 Twenty-four-hour tape may show intermittent non-sustained VT.
5 Exercise testing may show exercise-induced VT.
6 Other investigations will be targeted towards specific causes (e.g. cardiomyopathy screening; genetic screening etc.).

Williams syndrome – *see* Syndromes associated with cardiac
  abnormalities
Wolff–Parkinson–White (WPW) syndrome

WOLFF-PARKINSON-WHITE (WPW) SYNDROME

Wolff–Parkinson–White syndrome is a well known association of the following.
➤ Short PR interval:
  ➢ due to an accessory pathway bypassing the AV node
  ➢ therefore less time delay at the AV node.
➤ Ventricular pre-excitation:
  ➢ recognised as a delta wave on the ECG (an early upslope on the QRS)
  ➢ due to an accessory pathway bypassing the AV node
  ➢ this causes part of the ventricle to be stimulated before the rest
  ➢ as a result of the delta wave, the QRS complex will be wide
  ➢ Figure 6.65 shows a typical WPW ECG when in sinus rhythm.
➤ Paroxysmal tachycardia:
  ➢ usually a supraventricular tachycardia.

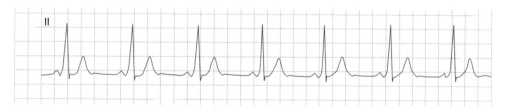

FIGURE 6.65 ECG demonstrating typical WPW with short PR interval, up-sloping
delta wave and widened QRS

WPW is present in around 0.3% of the population; many are asymptomatic.

WPW can be considered a congenital heart disease, as the accessory pathway
that bypasses the AV node is present from birth (i.e. it is an abnormal structure).
Figure 6.66 demonstrates this.

Often WPW is detected as an incidental finding when an ECG is performed
for other indications. However, children can also present with tachyarrhythmias.

Management of WPW will depend on the age and size of child, along with any
symptoms they are experiencing.

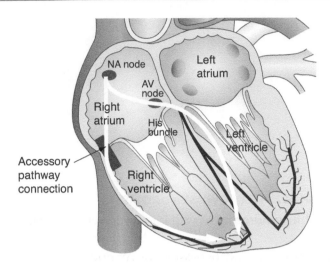

FIGURE 6.66 Accessory pathway in WPW syndrome, allowing electrical conduction to bypass the AV node – the pathway can be at any site left or right

Management of WPW includes the following.
➤ Treatment of the acute tachyarrhythmia (*see* Arrhythmias, SVT, VT and Cardioversion).
➤ Anti-arrhythmic drugs in infants (e.g. flecainide, amiodarone).
➤ Radiofrequency catheter ablation of the accessory pathway:
  ➤ usually only in older children
  ➤ may be performed in asymptomatic children if obvious WPW on ECG
  ➤ need to consider the risk : benefit ratio.

There is only a very small long-term risk of sudden cardiac death in people with WPW.

The most potential serious arrhythmia in people with WPW is atrial fibrillation; if this is present urgent DC cardioversion is needed. AF in WPW can be fatal as it can induce ventricular rates up to 400 bpm, causing rapid degeneration to ventricular fibrillation. It is rare in paediatric WPW, but can still occur.

Clinical features
> Asymptomatic
> Found on routine ECG
> Palpitations
> Supraventricular tachycardia (*see* page 176)

Investigations
1 ECG (Figure 6.65) demonstrates a short PR interval, wide QRS, and delta wave; it may demonstrate a SVT at times.
2 All basic imaging investigations are normal.

X

X-ray investigations – *see under* Investigations in suspected cardiac disease (chest X-ray and cardiac catheterisation)

CHAPTER 7

Hot topics: a quick reference guide

Ten common problems/diagnoses in paediatric cardiology
Incidence of congenital heart disease
Secondary hypertension
Syndromes with associated cardiac abnormalities
Heart failure
Syncope
Major causes of dilated cardiomyopathy
Long/short P-R interval
Long QT interval
Oligaemic lung fields
Plethoric lung fields

Ten common presenting complaints in paediatric cardiology
Syncope
Palpitations
Chest pain
Blue baby
Neonate with cardiogenic shock
Well child with murmur
Breathless infant
Breathless child
Bradycardic child
Child with hypertension

TEN COMMON PROBLEMS/DIAGNOSES IN PAEDIATRIC CARDIOLOGY

Incidence of congenital heart disease

Acyanotic

VSD	32%
PDA	12%
Pulmonary stenosis	8%
ASD	6%
Coarctation of the aorta	6%
Aortic stenosis	5%

Cyanotic

Tetralogy of Fallot	6%
TGA	5%

Secondary hypertension

Renal
➤ Renal scarring from urinary tract infection
➤ Renal artery stenosis
➤ Renal vein thrombosis
➤ Wilms' tumour

Cardiac
➤ Coarctation of the aorta

Endocrine
➤ Cushing's disease
➤ Primary hyperaldosteronism
➤ Phaeochromocytoma

Neurological
➤ Raised intracranial pressure (brain tumour)

Pharmacological
➤ Steroid use
➤ Recreational drug use

Miscellaneous
➤ Pain
➤ Anxiety

Syndromes with associated cardiac abnormalities

Down syndrome	VSD, AVSD
Edwards syndrome	VSD, double outlet right ventricle
DiGeorge syndrome	Truncus arteriosus, tetralogy of Fallot, VSD
Turner syndrome	Coarctation of the aorta
Noonan syndrome	Hypertrophic cardiomyopathy, ASD
	Pulmonary stenosis
Williams syndrome	Supravalvular aortic stenosis
	Peripheral pulmonary stenosis

Heart failure
➤ Hypoplastic left heart syndrome
➤ Critical coarctation of the aorta
➤ Critical aortic stenosis
➤ Interruption of the aortic arch
➤ Large VSD
➤ Large PDA (untreated) AVSD
➤ Cardiomyopathy

Syncope

Reflex (neurally mediated) syncope
➤ Vasovagal syncope (simple faint)
➤ Breath-holding attacks
➤ Reflex anoxic seizure
➤ Postural hypotension

Syncope of cardiac origin
➤ Cardiac arrhythmia
  ➤ complete heart block
  ➤ long QTc syndrome (causing polymorphic ventricular tachycardia)
  ➤ ventricular tachycardia (often monomorphic)
  ➤ sick sinus syndrome and SA node dysfunction
➤ Structural/functional heart defects
  ➤ aortic stenosis
  ➤ hypertrophic cardiomyopathy
  ➤ restrictive cardiomyopathy
➤ Pulmonary hypertension

Non-cardiac in origin
➤ Benign paroxysmal vertigo
➤ Migraine
➤ Fabricated or induced illness

Major causes of dilated cardiomyopathy

Major group	Main examples
Idiopathic	
Myocarditis	
Neuromuscular disease	*Duchenne muscular dystrophy*
	Becker's muscular dystrophy
	Myotonic dystrophy
Familial (genetic)	
Arrhythmia	*Recurrent or persistent tachycardia*
Inborn errors of metabolism	*Glycogen storage diseases, mucopolysaccharidoses, fatty acid oxidation defects*
Nutritional deficiency	*Vitamin B deficiency*
	Vitamin D deficiency
Toxin related	*Post-chemotherapy (especially with anthracyclines), iron overload*
Coronary artery disease	*ALCAPA*
	Myocardial infarction

Long/short P-R interval

Long P-R interval	Short P-R interval
Hyperkalaemia	Wolff–Parkinson–White syndrome
AVSD	Pompe disease
Hypothermia	Lown–Ganong–Levine syndrome
Duchenne muscular dystrophy	
Myocarditis	
Digoxin toxicity	

Long QT interval
➤ Familial/genetic
➤ Romano–Ward syndrome
➤ Jervell and Lange–Nielsen syndrome
➤ Hypokalaemia
➤ Hypomagnesaemia
➤ Hypothermia
➤ Hypocalcaemia
➤ Hypothyroidism
➤ Head injury
➤ Secondary to drugs: quinidine, tricyclic antidepressants, amiodarone.

Oligaemic lung fields

Any reduced pulmonary blood flow
- Tetralogy of Fallot
- Critical pulmonary stenosis
- Pulmonary hypertension
- Ebstein's anomaly

Plethoric lung fields

Any increased pulmonary blood flow
- TAPVD
- VSD
- AVSD
- PDA

TEN COMMON PRESENTING COMPLAINTS IN PAEDIATRIC CARDIOLOGY

Syncope

See Hot Topics, page 214

Cardiac syncope

➤ Arrhythmias (e.g. long QT, VT)

➤ Structural heart disease (e.g. HOCM, aortic stenosis)

➤ Pulmonary hypertension

Palpitations

➤ Sinus tachycardia

➤ Ventricular ectopic beats

➤ SVT

➤ VT

Chest pain

Non-cardiac (usually)

➤ Cardiac

➤ Pericarditis

➤ Aortic stenosis

➤ HOCM

➤ Coronary artery disease

Blue baby

Cardiac cyanosis

➤ Transposition of the great arteries

➤ Tetralogy of Fallot

➤ Tricuspid atresia

➤ Pulmonary atresia

➤ Truncus arteriosus

➤ Total anomalous pulmonary venous drainage

Non-cardiac cyanosis

➤ Persistent pulmonary hypertension of the newborn

➤ Sepsis

➤ Respiratory disease (e.g. pneumothorax, surfactant deficiency)

➤ Seizures

Neonate with cardiogenic shock

Duct-dependent lesions for systemic circulation

➤ Coarctation of the aorta

➤ Interrupted aortic arch

➤ Critical aortic stenosis
➤ Hypoplastic left heart

Well child with murmur

➤ Innocent murmur
➤ VSD
➤ ASD
➤ PDA
➤ Valve stenosis (mild)

Breathless infant

Cardiac
➤ Duct-dependent lesions
➤ Structural heart disease with heart failure (e.g. VSD)
➤ Cardiomyopathy
➤ Pericardial effusion
Non-cardiac

Breathless child

Cardiac
➤ Structural heart disease with heart failure (e.g. VSD)
➤ Cardiomyopathy
➤ Pericardial effusion
Non-cardiac

Bradycardic child

➤ Sinus bradycardia
➤ β-blockers
➤ Heart blocks

Child with hypertension

See Hot Topics, page 213 Coarctation of the aorta

Appendix

Blood pressure levels for boys by age and height centiles
Blood pressure levels for girls by age and height centiles
Paediatric ECG reference ranges
Cardiac catheterisation reference ranges

BLOOD PRESSURE LEVELS FOR BOYS BY AGE AND HEIGHT CENTILES

Age (Year)	BP Percentile ↓	Systolic BP (mmHg) ← Percentile of Height →							Diastolic BP (mmHg) ← Percentile of Height →						
		5th	10th	25th	50th	75th	90th	95th	5th	10th	25th	50th	75th	90th	95th
1	50th	80	81	83	85	87	88	89	34	35	36	37	38	39	39
	90th	94	95	97	99	100	102	103	49	50	51	52	53	53	54
	95th	98	99	101	103	104	106	106	54	54	55	56	57	58	58
	99th	105	106	108	110	112	113	114	61	62	63	64	65	66	66
2	50th	84	85	87	88	90	92	92	39	40	41	42	43	44	44
	90th	97	99	100	102	104	105	106	54	55	56	57	58	58	59
	95th	101	102	104	106	108	109	110	59	59	60	61	62	63	63
	99th	109	110	111	113	115	117	117	66	67	68	69	70	71	71
3	50th	86	87	89	91	93	94	95	44	44	45	46	47	48	48
	90th	100	101	103	105	107	108	109	59	59	60	61	62	63	63
	95th	104	105	107	109	110	112	113	63	63	64	65	66	67	67
	99th	111	112	114	116	118	119	120	71	71	72	73	74	75	75
4	50th	88	89	91	93	95	96	97	47	48	49	50	51	51	52
	90th	102	103	105	107	109	110	111	62	63	64	65	66	66	67
	95th	106	107	109	111	112	114	115	66	67	68	69	70	71	71
	99th	113	114	116	118	120	121	122	74	75	76	77	78	78	79
5	50th	90	91	93	95	96	98	98	50	51	52	53	54	55	55
	90th	104	105	106	108	110	111	112	65	66	67	68	69	69	70
	95th	108	109	110	112	114	115	116	69	70	71	72	73	74	74
	99th	115	116	118	120	121	123	123	77	78	79	80	81	81	82
6	50th	91	92	94	96	98	99	100	53	53	54	55	56	57	57
	90th	105	106	108	110	111	113	113	68	68	69	70	71	72	72
	95th	109	110	112	114	115	117	117	72	72	73	74	75	76	76
	99th	116	117	119	121	123	124	125	80	80	81	82	83	84	84
7	50th	92	94	95	97	99	100	101	55	55	56	57	58	59	59
	90th	106	107	109	111	113	114	115	70	70	71	72	73	74	74
	95th	110	111	113	115	117	118	119	74	74	75	76	77	78	78
	99th	117	118	120	122	124	125	126	82	82	83	84	85	86	86
8	50th	94	95	97	99	100	102	102	56	57	58	59	60	60	61
	90th	107	109	110	112	114	115	116	71	72	72	73	74	75	76
	95th	111	112	114	116	118	119	120	75	76	77	78	79	79	80
	99th	119	120	122	123	125	127	127	83	84	85	86	87	87	88
9	50th	95	96	98	100	102	103	104	57	58	59	60	61	61	62
	90th	109	110	112	114	115	117	118	72	73	74	75	76	76	77
	95th	113	114	116	118	119	121	121	76	77	78	79	80	81	81
	99th	120	121	123	125	127	128	129	84	85	86	87	88	88	89
10	50th	97	98	100	102	103	105	106	58	59	60	61	61	62	63
	90th	111	112	114	115	117	119	119	73	73	74	75	76	77	78
	95th	115	116	117	119	121	122	123	77	78	79	80	81	81	82
	99th	122	123	125	127	128	130	130	85	86	86	88	88	89	90

Age (Year)	BP Percentile ↓	Systolic BP (mmHg) ← Percentile of Height →							Diastolic BP (mmHg) ← Percentile of Height →						
		5th	10th	25th	50th	75th	90th	95th	5th	10th	25th	50th	75th	90th	95th
11	50th	99	100	102	104	105	107	107	59	59	60	61	62	63	63
	90th	113	114	115	117	119	120	121	74	74	75	76	77	78	78
	95th	117	118	119	121	123	124	125	78	78	79	80	81	82	82
	99th	124	125	127	129	130	132	132	86	86	87	88	89	90	90
12	50th	101	102	104	106	108	109	110	59	60	61	62	63	63	64
	90th	115	116	118	120	121	123	123	74	75	75	76	77	78	79
	95th	119	120	122	123	125	127	127	78	79	80	81	82	82	83
	99th	126	127	129	131	133	134	135	86	87	88	89	90	90	91
13	50th	104	105	106	108	110	111	112	60	60	61	62	63	64	64
	90th	117	118	120	122	124	125	126	75	75	76	77	78	79	79
	95th	121	122	124	126	128	129	130	79	79	80	81	82	83	83
	99th	128	130	131	133	135	136	137	87	87	88	89	90	91	91
14	50th	106	107	109	111	113	114	115	60	61	62	63	64	65	65
	90th	120	121	123	125	126	128	128	75	76	77	78	79	79	80
	95th	124	125	127	128	130	132	132	80	80	81	82	83	84	84
	99th	131	132	134	136	138	139	140	87	88	89	90	91	92	92
15	50th	109	110	112	113	115	117	117	61	62	63	64	65	66	66
	90th	122	124	125	127	129	130	131	76	77	78	79	80	80	81
	95th	126	127	129	131	133	134	135	81	81	82	83	84	85	85
	99th	134	135	136	138	140	142	142	88	89	90	91	92	93	93
16	50th	111	112	114	116	118	119	120	63	63	64	65	66	67	67
	90th	125	126	128	130	131	133	134	78	78	79	80	81	82	82
	95th	129	130	132	134	135	137	137	82	83	83	84	85	86	87
	99th	136	137	139	141	143	144	145	90	90	91	92	93	94	94
17	50th	114	115	116	118	120	121	122	65	66	66	67	68	69	70
	90th	127	128	130	132	134	135	136	80	80	81	82	83	84	84
	95th	131	132	134	136	138	139	140	84	85	86	87	87	88	89
	99th	139	140	141	143	145	146	147	92	93	93	94	95	96	97

BP, blood pressure

* The 90th percentile is 1.28 SD, 95th percentile is 1.645 SD, and the 99th percentile is 2.326 SD over the mean.

BLOOD PRESSURE LEVELS FOR GIRLS BY AGE AND HEIGHT CENTILES

Age (Year)	BP Percentile ↓	Systolic BP (mmHg) ← Percentile of Height →							Diastolic BP (mmHg) ← Percentile of Height →						
		5th	10th	25th	50th	75th	90th	95th	5th	10th	25th	50th	75th	90th	95th
1	50th	83	84	85	86	88	89	90	38	39	39	40	41	41	42
	90th	97	97	98	100	101	102	103	52	53	53	54	55	55	56
	95th	100	101	102	104	105	106	107	56	57	57	58	59	59	60
	99th	108	108	109	111	112	113	114	64	64	65	65	66	67	67
2	50th	85	85	87	88	89	91	91	43	44	44	45	46	46	47
	90th	98	99	100	101	103	104	105	57	58	58	59	60	61	61
	95th	102	103	104	105	107	108	109	61	62	62	63	64	65	65
	99th	109	110	111	112	114	115	116	69	69	70	70	71	72	72
3	50th	86	87	88	89	91	92	93	47	48	48	49	50	50	51
	90th	100	100	102	103	104	106	106	61	62	62	63	64	64	65
	95th	104	104	105	107	108	109	110	65	66	66	67	68	68	69
	99th	111	111	113	114	115	116	117	73	73	74	74	75	76	76
4	50th	88	88	90	91	92	94	94	50	50	51	52	52	53	54
	90th	101	102	103	104	106	107	108	64	64	65	66	67	67	68
	95th	105	106	107	108	110	111	112	68	68	69	70	71	71	72
	99th	112	113	114	115	117	118	119	76	76	76	77	78	79	79
5	50th	89	90	91	93	94	95	96	52	53	53	54	55	55	56
	90th	103	103	105	106	107	109	109	66	67	67	68	69	69	70
	95th	107	107	108	110	111	112	113	70	71	71	72	73	73	74
	99th	114	114	116	117	118	120	120	78	78	79	79	80	81	81
6	50th	91	92	93	94	96	97	98	54	54	55	56	56	57	58
	90th	104	105	106	108	109	110	111	68	68	69	70	70	71	72
	95th	108	109	110	111	113	114	115	72	72	73	74	74	75	76
	99th	115	116	117	119	120	121	122	80	80	80	81	82	83	83
7	50th	93	93	95	96	97	99	99	55	56	56	57	58	58	59
	90th	106	107	108	109	111	112	113	69	70	70	71	72	72	73
	95th	110	111	112	113	115	116	116	73	74	74	75	76	76	77
	99th	117	118	119	120	122	123	124	81	81	82	82	83	84	84
8	50th	95	95	96	98	99	100	101	57	57	57	58	59	60	60
	90th	108	109	110	111	113	114	114	71	71	71	72	73	74	74
	95th	112	112	114	115	116	118	118	75	75	75	76	77	78	78
	99th	119	120	121	122	123	125	125	82	82	83	83	84	85	86
9	50th	96	97	98	100	101	102	103	58	58	58	59	60	61	61
	90th	110	110	112	113	114	116	116	72	72	72	73	74	75	75
	95th	114	114	115	117	118	119	120	76	76	76	77	78	79	79
	99th	121	121	123	124	125	127	127	83	83	84	84	85	86	87
10	50th	98	99	100	102	103	104	105	59	59	59	60	61	62	62
	90th	112	112	114	115	116	118	118	73	73	73	74	75	76	76
	95th	116	116	117	119	120	121	122	77	77	77	78	79	80	80
	99th	123	123	125	126	127	129	129	84	84	85	86	86	87	88

Age (Year)	BP Percentile ↓	Systolic BP (mmHg)							Diastolic BP (mmHg)						
		← Percentile of Height →							← Percentile of Height →						
		5th	10th	25th	50th	75th	90th	95th	5th	10th	25th	50th	75th	90th	95th
11	50th	100	101	102	103	105	106	107	60	60	60	61	62	63	63
	90th	114	114	116	117	118	119	120	74	74	74	75	76	77	77
	95th	118	118	119	121	122	123	124	78	78	78	79	80	81	81
	99th	125	125	126	128	129	130	131	85	85	86	87	87	88	89
12	50th	102	103	104	105	107	108	109	61	61	61	62	63	64	64
	90th	116	116	117	119	120	121	122	75	75	75	76	77	78	78
	95th	119	120	121	123	124	125	126	79	79	79	80	81	82	82
	99th	127	127	128	130	131	132	133	86	86	87	88	88	89	90
13	50th	104	105	106	107	109	110	110	62	62	62	63	64	65	65
	90th	117	118	119	121	122	123	124	76	76	76	77	78	79	79
	95th	121	122	123	124	126	127	128	80	80	80	81	82	83	83
	99th	128	129	130	132	133	134	135	87	87	88	89	89	90	91
14	50th	106	106	107	109	110	111	112	63	63	63	64	65	66	66
	90th	119	120	121	122	124	125	125	77	77	77	78	79	80	80
	95th	123	123	125	126	127	129	129	81	81	81	82	83	84	84
	99th	130	131	132	133	135	136	136	88	88	89	90	90	91	92
15	50th	107	108	109	110	111	113	113	64	64	64	65	66	67	67
	90th	120	121	122	123	125	126	127	78	78	78	79	80	81	81
	95th	124	125	126	127	129	130	131	82	82	82	83	84	85	85
	99th	131	132	133	134	136	137	138	89	89	90	91	91	92	93
16	50th	108	108	110	111	112	114	114	64	64	65	66	66	67	68
	90th	121	122	123	124	126	127	128	78	78	79	80	81	81	82
	95th	125	126	127	128	130	131	132	82	82	83	84	85	85	86
	99th	132	133	134	135	137	138	139	90	90	90	91	92	93	93
17	50th	108	109	110	111	113	114	115	64	65	65	66	67	67	68
	90th	122	122	123	125	126	127	128	78	79	79	80	81	81	82
	95th	125	126	127	129	130	131	132	82	83	83	84	85	85	86
	99th	133	133	134	136	137	138	139	90	90	91	91	92	93	93

BP, blood pressure

* The 90th percentile is 1.28 SD, 95th percentile is 1.645 SD, and the 99th percentile is 2.326 SD over the mean.

Paediatric BP charts obtained from the National Heart Lung and Blood Institute's 2004 guidelines 'High Blood Pressure in Children & Adolescence'. Available at: www.nhlbi.nih.gov/guidelines/hypertension/child_tbl.pdf

PAEDIATRIC ECG REFERENCE RANGES

Neonatal reference ranges 1

Age	Heart Rate (Beats per min)	Frontal Plane QRS Axis (Degrees)	PR Interval (Seconds)	QRS Duration (Seconds)	R Amplitude in V1 (mm)	R Amplitude in V6 (mm)
0–1 day	93–154	+59 to +192	0.08–0.16	0.02–0.08	5–26	0–11
1–3 days	91–159	+64 to +197	0.08–0.14	0.02–0.07	5–27	0–12
3–7 days	90–166	+77 to +187	0.08–0.14	0.02–0.07	3–24	0.5–12
7–30 days	107–182	+65 to +160	0.07–0.14	0.02–0.08	3–21.5	2.5–16
1–3 months	121–179	+31 to +114	0.07–0.13	0.02–0.08	3–18.5	5–21

Paediatric reference ranges 2

Age	Heart Rate (Beats per min)	Frontal Plane QRS Axis (Degrees)	PR Interval (Seconds)	QRS Duration (Seconds)	R Amplitude in V1 (mm)	R Amplitude in V6 (mm)
3–5 months	105–185	0 to +135	0.08–0.15	0.03–0.08	3–20	6–22
6–11 months	110–170	0 to +135	0.07–0.16	0.03–0.08	2–20	6–23
1–2 years	90–165	0 to +110	0.08–0.16	0.03–0.08	2–18	4–24
3–4 years	70–140	0 to +110	0.09–0.17	0.04–0.08	1–18	4–24
5–7 years	65–140	0 to +110	0.09–0.17	0.04–0.08	0.5–14	4–26
8–11 years	60–130	−15 to +110	0.09–0.17	0.04–0.09	0–14	4–25
12–15 years	65–130	−15 to +110	0.09–0.18	0.04–0.09	0–14	4–25

Adult reference ranges

Age	Heart Rate (Beats per min)	Frontal Plane QRS Axis (Degrees)	PR Interval (Seconds)	QRS Duration (Seconds)	R Amplitude in V1 (mm)	R Amplitude in V6 (mm)
>16 years	60–100	−30 to +90	0.12–0.20	0.06–0.10	0–14	4–20

1 Schwartz PJ, Garson A, Paul T, *et al*. Guidelines for the interpretation of the neonatal electrocardiogram. *Eur Heart J.* 2002; **23**: 1329–44.

2 Sharieff GQ, Rao SO. The pediatric ECG. *Emerg Med Clin North Am.* 2006; **24**:196.

CARDIAC CATHETERISATION REFERENCE RANGES

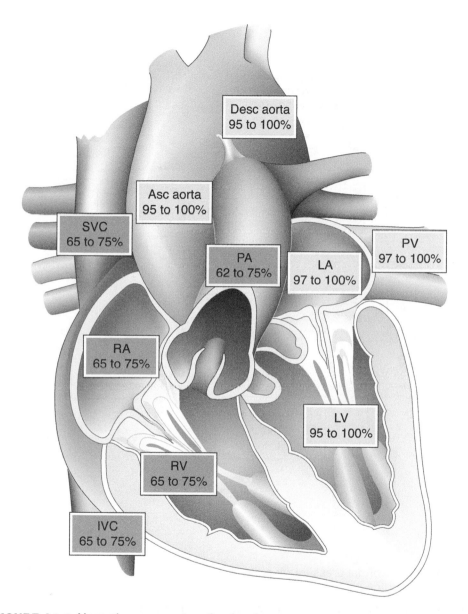

FIGURE A1.1 Normal oxygen saturation levels

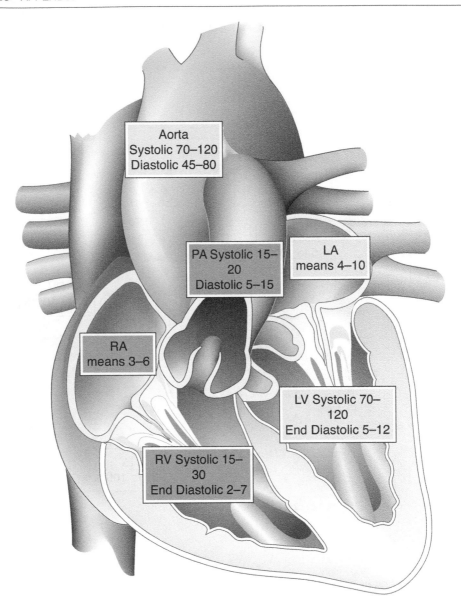

FIGURE A1.2 Normal pressure recordings

All pressure measurements quoted are recorded in mmHg.

Note that the pressures in the left ventricle and aorta are age dependent. The aortic pressure should represent the blood pressure obtained in the arm. Please see the centile charts for BP for normal values.

Glossary

ABG	arterial blood gases
ABPM	ambulatory blood pressure monitoring
ACE	angiotensin-converting enzyme
AD	autosomal dominant
A&E	Accident & Emergency
AF	atrial fibrillation
ALCAPA	anomalous left coronary artery from the pulmonary artery
ANCA	anti-neutrophil cytoplasmic antibodies
APLS	advanced paediatric life support
AR	aortic regurgitation
AR	autosomal recessive
AS	aortic stenosis
ASD	atrial septal defect
ASOT	anti-streptolysin O titre
AV	atrioventricular
AVN	atrioventricular node
AVNRT	atrioventricular nodal re-entry tachycardia
AVRT	atrioventricular re-entry tachycardia
AVSD	atrioventricular septal defect
BBB	blood–brain barrier
BC	blood culture
BiVAD	biventricular assist device
BP	blood pressure
BT shunt	Blalock–Taussig shunt
CAA	coronary artery aneurysm
CAVSD	complete atrioventricular septal defect
CF	cystic fibrosis
cAMP	cyclic adenosine monophosphate
cGMP	cyclic guanosine monophosphate
CHARGE	coloboma, heart disease, choanal atresia, retarded growth & development, genital hypoplasia, ear abnormalities
CHD	congenital heart disease
CK	creatine kinase
CMRI	cardiac magnetic resonance imaging
CMV	cytomegalovirus
CNS	central nervous system

CO	cardiac output
CPB	cardiopulmonary bypass surgery
CPR	cardiopulmonary resuscitation
CRP	C reactive protein
CSF	cerebrospinal fluid
CT	computed tomography
CXR	chest X-ray
DC	direct current
DCM	dilated cardiomyopathy
DILV	double inlet left ventricle
DMD	Duchenne muscular dystrophy
DORV	double outlet right ventricle
DS	Down syndrome
D&V	diarrhoea & vomiting
ECG	electrocardiogram
Echo	echocardiography
ECMO	extracorporeal membrane oxygenation
ESM	ejection systolic murmur
ESR	erythrocyte sedimentation rate
ETT	endotracheal tube
FBC	full blood count
FiO_2	fractional inspired oxygen
FISH	fluorescent in situ hybridisation
GA	general anaesthesia
GI	gastrointestinal
GP	general practitioner
GSD	glycogen storage disease
GTN	glyceryl trinitrate
Hb	haemoglobin
HCM	hypertrophic cardiomyopathy
HFO	high-frequency oscillation
HLHS	hypoplastic left heart syndrome
HOCM	hypertrophic obstructive cardiomyopathy
HR	heart rate
IAA	interrupted aortic arch
IBD	inflammatory bowel disease
ICD	implantable cardioverter defibrillator
IE	infective endocarditis
IM	intramuscular
IV	intravenous
IVC	inferior vena cava
IVIG	intravenous immunoglobulin
JIA	juvenile idiopathic arthritis

JVP	jugular venous pressure
KD	Kawasaki disease
LAD	left axis deviation
LBBB	left bundle branch block
LCA	left coronary artery
LFT	liver function test
LMBT shunt	left modified Blalock–Taussig shunt
LP	lumbar puncture
LSE	left sternal edge
LV	left ventricle
LVAD	left ventricular assist device
LVH	left ventricular hypertrophy
LVOT	left ventricular outflow tract
MAPCAs	major aortopulmonary collateral arteries
MAS	meconium aspiration syndrome
MCV	mean corpuscular volume
MEGX	monoethylglycinexylidide
MI	myocardial infarction
MMR	measles, mumps, rubella
MPA	main pulmonary artery
MPS	mucopolysaccharidosis
MR	mitral regurgitation
MRI	magnetic resonance imaging
MS	mitral stenosis
NICE	National Institute for Health and Clinical Excellence
NLS	neonatal life support
NO	nitric oxide
NSAID	non-steroidal anti-inflammatory drug
OI	oxygenation index
PA	pulmonary artery
PA	pulmonary atresia
$PaCO_2$	arterial carbon dioxide tension
PAPVD	partial anomalous pulmonary venous drainage
PCOS	polycystic ovarian syndrome
PDA	patent ductus arteriosus
PEEP	positive end-expiratory pressure
PFO	patent foramen ovale
PH	pulmonary hypertension
PICU	Paediatric Intensive Care Unit
PJRT	permanent junctional re-entry tachycardia
PO_2	partial pressure oxygen
PPHN	persistent pulmonary hypertension of the newborn
PROM	prolonged rupture of membranes

PS	pulmonary stenosis
PTH	parathyroid hormone
PVR	pulmonary vascular resistance
RA	right atrium
RAD	right axis deviation
RBBB	right bundle branch block
RCPCH	Royal College of Paediatrics and Child Health
RMBT shunt	right modified Blalock–Taussig shunt
RSE	right sternal edge
RSV	respiratory syncytial virus
RV	right ventricle
RVOT	right ventricle outflow tract
SA	sinoatrial
SAN	sinoatrial node
SaO_2	arterial oxygen saturation
SCBU	Special Care Baby Unit
SLE	systemic lupus erythematosus
SMA	spinal muscular atrophy
SV	stroke volume
SVC	superior vena cava
SVT	supraventricular tachycardia
TAPVC	total anomalous pulmonary venous connection
TAPVD	total anomalous pulmonary venous drainage
TCPC	total cavopulmonary connection
TFT	thyroid function test
TGA	transposition of the great arteries
TOE	transoesophageal echocardiogram
ToF	tetralogy of Fallot
TOF	tracheo-oesophageal fistula
TSH	thyroid stimulating hormone
U&Es	urea & electrolytes
URTI	upper respiratory tract infection
UTI	urinary tract infection
UVC	umbilical venous catheter
VA	venoarterial
VACTERL	vertebral, anal, cardiac, trachea-oesophageal fistula, ears, renal, limb abnormalities
VAD	ventricular assist device
VF	ventricular fibrillation
VI	ventilation index
VSD	ventricular septal defect
VT	ventricular tachycardia
VV	venovenous

WBC	white blood cell
WPW	Wolff–Parkinson–White syndrome
XD	X-linked dominant
XR	X-linked recessive

Index

Entries in **bold** refer to figures and tables.

α-agonists 26
α-blockers 34
Acanthosis nigricans 121
ACE (angiotensin converting
  enzyme) inhibitors 27
    and cardiomyopathy 87
    drug interactions of 34
    and heart failure 77, 85
    in pre-transplant patients
    194
    and VSD 205
acetazolamide 27
Actinobacillus 125
Addison's disease 30, 35
adenosine 28, 177–9
adrenaline 28
    and cardiac conduction 14
    and heart rate 24
    inotropic effect of 22, 26
Alagille syndrome 166, 176,
  181
ALCAPA (anomalous left
  coronary artery from the
  pulmonary artery) 66–7
    and heart structure 14
    and mitral regurgitation 137
    and ST elevation 53–4
alcohol 28, 32–3, 96
aldosterone antagonists 27
amiodarone 28–9
    anti-arrhythmic effect of 27
    and cardioversion 92
    drug interactions of 32
    and long QT 215
    and VT 208
anaemia 85, 97, 127–8
anaesthesia, general 33, 61
anagrelide 33
anaphylaxis 28, 33
anastomosis 94
angina 28–9, 31, 35, 67
angiography, coronary 67,
  194
anomaly scan 110
anterior chest wall 11
anti-arrhythmic medications 24,
  27–8, 35, 168, 178, 210
antibacterials 32
antibiotics
    and infective endocarditis
    126
    and long QT 168

antidepressants 28–9, 35, 207,
  215
antihypertensive medications
  95, 121
anxiety 23, 120, 127, 213
aorta, dilated 68, 82
aortic atresia 122
aortic coarctation 93–5, **93**
    as acyanotic 65–6
    antenatal detection of 111
    and AVSD 77
    and bicuspid valves 14, 82
    and duct-dependent
    circulation 102
    and Edwards syndrome 182
    and femoral pulse 37
    and hypertension 120
    and Patau syndrome 184
    and phenylketonuria 96
    repair of 91
    and Shone's Complex 138
    and TGA 196
    and Turner syndrome 184,
    214
aortic dissection 153, 182–3
aortic knuckle 68
aortic root 67–9, 71
aortic stenosis 69–70
    as acyanotic 65–6
    and bicuspid aortic valve
    82
    and bundle branch block 50
    critical 69, 102, 214
    and exercise testing 62
    and HLHS 122
    and syncope 179
    and thrills 38
    and ventricular hypertrophy
    52
    and Williams syndrome 214
aortic valve
    congenitally abnormal 67,
    69
    damaged 67
    insufficiency 72
    normal function of **68**
    replacement of 68, 70, 82
    structure of 14
APLS (advanced paediatric life
  support) 94
    algorithm 178, 207
    guidelines 102

apnoea 34
AR (aortic regurgitation) 67–9,
  82, 137, 182–3
arrhythmias 70, **71**
    acquired 65
    cardiac output in 19
    and cardiomyopathy 87, 89,
    215
    and cardioversion 91
    and chest X-ray 59
    and Ebstein's anomaly 105
    and ECG 51, 61
    and Eisenmenger syndrome
    109
    exercise-induced 62
    fetal 111
    and Fontan procedure 112
    and long QT 170
    and medications 31
    and Mustard procedure 143
    and myocarditis 145
    risk of 15
    sinus 45, 55
    supraventricular 28, 32
    and syncope 179
    ventricular 33
    in WPW 210
arterial switch procedure 71–2,
  74, 91, 142, 198
ascites 30, 34, 86
ASD (atrial septal defect) 72–6
    definition of 13
    as acyanotic 65
    and axis deviation 48
    and bundle branch blocks
    50
    and echocardiograms 61
    and Eisenmenger syndrome
    108
    and Noonan syndrome
    214
    and PAPVD 193
    primum 73–6, **75**, 78–9
    secundum 73–4, **74**, 76
    and TGA 196
    and truncus arteriosus 201
asplenia syndrome 131
asthma 28–9, 160
asystole 29, 35
atenolol 27, 29, 169
atrial arrhythmias 19, 71, 76,
  177

atrial fibrillation
and medications 28, 31–2
and mitral regurgitation 137
and mitral stenosis 138
in WPW 210
atrial flutter 31, 45, 73, 178
atrial hypertrophy
left 49–50, 139
right 49, 105, 160
atrial tachycardia 45, 49, 73, 176
atropine 24, 29
auscultation 36, 38, 197, 203
AV (atrioventricular) block 32,
35, 117–18
AV (atrioventricular) fistula 108
AV (atrioventricular) re-entry
tachycardia 49, 176
AVN (atrioventricular node)
in cardiac conduction 14–15,
23
damage to 119
medications acting on 28–9,
35
in SVT 176–7
and WPW 209
AVSD (atrioventricular septal
defect) 77–9
definition of 13
and axis deviation 48
complete 60, 79
and CPB 91
and Eisenmenger syndrome
108
and Glenn shunt 115
and heart block 116
and lung fields 216
and PA bands 162
partial 48, 73–4, **75**, 77–9,
78
and PPHN 158
and PR interval 54, 215
types of **79**
axis deviation
and ASD 76
and AVSD 79
left 48, 52, 68, 101, 183
right 48, 52, 188
types of 48

β-blockers
anti-arrhythmic effect of 27
and bradycardia 218
and cardiomyopathy 144
drug interactions of 28–9,
32–5
and heart failure 85
and heart rate 24
and hypertension 95
inotropic effect of 23
and long QT 208
in pre-transplant patients
194
balloon atrial septostomy 71,
101–2, 165, 171, **172**, 198

balloon dilatation 138, 167
balloon valvuloplasty 70, 82
Bartter syndrome 34
Bazett's formula 55, 168
Becker's muscular dystrophy 215
Beck's Triad 155
bendroflumethiazide 26
benign paroxysmal vertigo 181,
214
Berlin Heart 80–1, 85, 87, 106,
194
Best of Five questions 3
bicuspid aortic valve 67, 81–2,
81
and coarctation 93
and Edwards syndrome 182
and heart sounds 142
and Patau syndrome 184
and Turner sydnrome 184
birth asphyxia 157
BiVAD (biventricular assist
device) 80–1, **80**
biventricular hypertrophy 152,
197, 201, 205
biventricular pacing 85
Blalock–Taussig (BT) shunt
82–3, **83**
and DORV 101
and duct-dependent
circulation 102
as non-bypass 91
and Norwood procedure
146–7
and pulmonary atresia 165
and tetralogy of Fallot 189
and tricuspid 199
blood–brain barrier (BBB) 29,
32
blood gas 86, 90, 130
blue babies 97, 105, 217
bosentan 30, 161
BP (blood pressure)
and aortic stenosis 70
and cardiac function 22
and cardiac output 21
control of 24, **25**
in exercise testing 62
and hypertension 119
ranges for **219–23**
brachiofemoral delay 95
bradycardia 218
definition of 45, 70
and heart block 116, 118
and medications 29, 33–5
breast feeding 29–30, 33
bronchiectasis 131
bronchiolitis 84, 106, 115, 149
Bruce protocol 61
Brugada syndrome 32, 50, 53,
207
bumetanide 26
bundle branch blocks 119
and axis deviation 48
and QRS complex 50–1

risk of 15
see also LBBB; RBBB

calcium channel blockers 23,
27, 31, 34–5
cAMP (cyclic adenosine
monophosphate) 28, 33
captopril 27, 30, 85
carbonic anhydrase inhibitors
27
cardiac anatomy 10–11, 130; see
also heart, structure of
cardiac arrest
and cardiac tamponade 154
and cardioversion 92
and ECMO 106
and medications 28, 34
and VT 206–8
cardiac catheterisation
and aortic coarctation 94
diagnostic, see diagnostic
catheterisation
and PDA 152
and PFO 73
and pulmonary hypotension
161
and Rashkind procedure 171
reference ranges for **225–6**
and valvuloplasty 70
and VSD 205
cardiac conduction system
14–15, **15**, 23
cardiac cycle 18–20, **19–20**, 92
cardiac enzymes 67, 145
cardiac failure
and aortic coarctation 94
and ASD 76
and AVSD 77, 79
and cardiac output 21
and cardiomyopathy 86, 89
causes of **84–5**
congestive, see congestive
heart failure
and DORV 101
and ECMO 106
and Eisenmenger syndrome
109
and IAA 130
infant 203
and Kawasaki disease 134
and medications 30–2, 34–5
and mitral stenosis 139
and myocarditis 144
right-sided 38, 161
severe 31, 81, 86
signs of 40
and TAPVD 192
and truncus arteriosus 201
cardiac function, assessment of
21–2
cardiac glycosides 26, 31
cardiac pharmacology 26–7
cardiac physiology 17
cardiac rejection 194–5

cardiac surgery
  and medications 33–4
  and PR interval 54
  and ST elevation 53
  and VT 207
cardiac tamponade 154–5
cardiac transplantation
  and Berlin Heart 80–1
  and cardiac failure 85
  and cardiomyopathy 87, 89
  and ECMO 106
  and HLHS 122
  and myocarditis 144
cardiogenic shock
  and aortic coarctation 94
  and duct-dependent
    circulation 102–3
  and IAA 129–30
  and LVOT obstruction 66
  and medications 29, 31
  and myocarditis 145
  and TAPVD 192
  and tricuspid atresia 200
  and truncus arteriosus 201
cardiology
  common presenting
    complaints 217–18
  investigations in 57
cardiomegaly
  and aortic regurgitation 68
  and AVSD 79
  and cardiac rejection 195
  and congenital heart disease
    95
  and heart failure 86
  and hypertension 121
  and hypoplastic left heart
    123
  and myocarditis 144
  and PDA 152
  and pulmonary stenosis
    167
Cardiomemo 61, 179
cardiomyopathy 86–9
  acquired 65
  and ALCAPA 67
  and atrial hypertrophy 49
  and Berlin Heart 81
  dilated, see dilated
    cardiomyopathy
  and heart transplantation
    144, 193
  inotropic effects of 23
  and mitral regurgitation 137
  and pericardial effusion 153
  screening for 85–6, 89–90,
    208
  and ST segments 54
  and T waves 53
  and ventricular hypertrophy
    52
  and VT 207
cardiovascular system,
  examination of 36, 40

cardioversion 84, 91–3, 177,
  178, 208, 210
carditis, acute 168
carotid sinus massage 178
carvedilol 85
case histories 4–5
catecholamines 14, 24, 31
CAVSD (complete
  atrioventricular septal defects)
  13, 48, 77, **78**
cerebral anoxia, transient 179
cerebral arteriovenous
  malformations 158
cerebrovascular accidents 187–8
cervical lymphadenopathy
  133–4
cGMP (cyclic guanosine
  monophosphate) 33–4
CHARGE syndrome 129, 176,
  181
chest pain
  and aortic stenosis 70
  and Eisenmenger syndrome
    109
  in exercise testing 62
  and myocarditis 145
  precordial 161
  retrosternal 155
  and SVT 179
chest walls, thin 60, 127
chlorothiazide 30, 85
ciliary dyskinesia 131
circulation
  duct-dependent 96, 101–3,
    122, 163, 201
  fetal 15–17, 17
  mixing of blood between 196
  pulmonary and systemic 12
cleft palate 181–4
clubbing 37, 105, 109
CO (cardiac output)
  and aortic coarctation 94
  and arrhythmia 19
  calculation of 21
  and fluid resuscitation 23
  low 33, 139, 155
  medications and 31, 35
  and VT 207
cocaine 96, 101
conduction system 11, 14–15,
  116, 119
congenital diaphragmatic hernia
  158, 182
congenital heart disease (CHD)
  acyanotic 65–6
  antenatal diagnosis of 110
  and antibiotics 126
  and cardiomyopathy 87
  common 96
  complex 59, 193
  cyanotic 82, 97–8, 101, 162
  and dextrocardia 130
  and Eisenmenger syndrome
    107–8

  and endocarditis 124
  exercise tolerance in 62
  incidence of 213
  murmurs in 140
  and polycythaemia 37
  and pulmonary hypertension
    160
  and Rashkind procedure 171
congestive heart failure
  and acyanotic CHD 65
  and ALCAPA 67
  and endocarditis 125
  and medications 32–3
  and myocarditis 145
  and PDA 152
  and pulmonary stenosis 167
  and rheumatic fever 175
  and tetralogy of Fallot 188
conjunctival injection 133
constipation 29, 35
coronary arteries 14, 66–7, **66**,
  71–2, 198, 200
  aneurysms of, see Kawasaki
    disease
coronary artery disease 137, 194
cough 30, 127, 155
coxsackie virus 153
CPB (cardiopulmonary bypass)
  84, 90–1, **91**
CPR (cardiopulmonary
  resuscitation) 28–9, 32
Cushing's disease 120, 213
CXR (chest X-ray)
  and ALCAPA 67
  and aortic coarctation 95
  and aortic regurgitation 68
  and aortic stenosis 70
  and ASD 75
  and AVSD 79
  and cardiac defects 58–9
  and cardiac rejection 195
  and cardiomyopathy 89
  and DORV 101
  and Ebstein's anomaly 105
  and Eisenmenger syndrome
    109
  findings from 59
  and heart failure 86
  and hypertension 121
  and hypoplastic left heart
    123
  and IAA 130
  and isomerism defects 131
  and mitral stenosis 139
  and myocarditis 144
  and pericardial effusion 155
  and PPHN 158
  and pulmonary atresia 165
  and pulmonary hypertension
    160
  and pulmonary stenosis 167
  summary of 58
  and TAPVD 192
  and TGA 197

CXR (*continued*)
    and tricuspid atresia 200
    and truncus arteriosus 201
    and VSD 206
cyanosis
    central 97
    and duct-dependent
      circulation 102
    and Ebstein's anomaly 105
    and Eisenmenger syndrome
      109
    and Glenn shunt 115
    and hypoplastic left heart
      123
    in inspection 36–7
    neonatal 97, 100, 165
    peripheral 97
    and pulmonary hypotension
      161
    and pulmonary stenosis 167
    and TAPVD 192
    and tetralogy of Fallot 186–7,
      189
    and TGA 197–8
    and tricuspid atresia
      198–200
    and truncus arteriosus 201
cystic fibrosis 160

D-receptor agonists 26
Danon disease 88
data interpretation 5
deafness, *see* hearing loss
defibrillators 92, 208
delta waves 51, 54, 209–10
demographic data 41–3
depolarisation, spontaneous
    rate of 23
dextrocardia 130–1
    and apex beats 38
    and axis deviation 48
    and P waves 49
dextroposition 130
diabetes 32, 96
    maternal 101, 110, 198, 201
diabetic nephropathy 30
diagnostic catheterisation 62–3
    and aortic stenosis 70
    and DORV 101
    and mitral stenosis 139
    and pulmonary atresia 165
    and TAPVD 192
    and truncus arteriosus 202
    and VSD 206
diarrhoea 31, 115
diastolic murmurs 39, 69, 109,
    139–40, 142, 206
DiGeorge syndrome 129–30,
    164, 166, 176, 181, 201–2
digitalis poisoning 31–2
digoxin 31
    drug interactions of 29, 32
    and heart failure 85
    inotropic effect of 26

and ST segments 54
and T waves **53**
and VT 207
digoxin toxicity 54, 116–17, 215
dilated cardiomyopathy 87, **88**
    major causes of 215
    and myocarditis 144–5
    and Q waves 52
diltiazem 27
DILV (double inlet left
    ventricle) 99–100, **99**, 115,
    162
Diploma in Child Health
    (DCH) 2
diuretics
    in cardiac pharmacology
      26–7, 30–1
    and cardiomyopathy 87,
      144
    and heart failure 77, 85
    and PDA 152
    in pre-transplant patients
      194
    and pulmonary hypertension
      161
    and tricuspid atresia 199
    and truncus arteriosus 201
    and VSD 205
dizziness 28, 31–2, 62, 155, 179
dobutamine 31
    and cardiomyopathy 87
    and heart failure 85
    inotropic effect of 22, 26
    in pre-transplant patients
      194
dopamine 31
    and heart failure 85
    inotropic effect of 22, 26
    and noradrenaline 33
DORV (double outlet right
    ventricle) 100–1, **100**, 173,
    181, 214
Down syndrome 176, 181, 214
    antenatal detection of 111
    and AVSD 73, 77, 79
    and CHD 96
    and VSD 203
drug use
    and hypertension 120
    maternal 96, 111
drugs, names of 5
Duchenne muscular dystrophy
    215
ductus arteriosus 16, 34, 93–4,
    150–1, 198
ductus venosus 16
Duke's criteria 126
dyspnoea
    and ASD 76
    and Eisenmenger syndrome
      109
    and medications 28, 32
    and myocarditis 145
    paroxysmal nocturnal 85

and pulmonary hypertension
    161
and pulmonary stenosis 167
and tetralogy of Fallot 189

Ebstein's anomaly 104–5, **104**
    and atrial hypertrophy 49
    and axis deviation 48
    and Glenn shunt 115
    and lithium 96
    and lung fields 216
    and PPHN 158
    and valve offset 13
ECG (electrocardiogram)
    and ALCAPA 67
    ambulatory recordings 61
    and aortic coarctation 95
    and aortic regurgitation 68
    and aortic stenosis 70
    and ASD 76
    and AVSD 79
    and cardiac cycle **20**
    and cardiac rejection 195
    and cardiomyopathy 89
    and cardioversion 92
    and dextrocardia 131
    and DORV 101
    and Ebstein's anomaly 105
    in examination 5
    forming opinion on 55
    heart block on 118
    and heart failure 86
    and hypertension 121
    and hypoplastic left heart
      123
    interpretation of 41, **42–3**
    and Kawasaki disease 134
    and Klippel–Feil sequence
      183
    lead-placement landmarks
      58
    and long QT syndrome **170**
    and mitral stenosis 139
    and myocarditis 144
    and pericardial effusion 155
    and pericarditis **156**
    placement of leads 11
    and pulmonary atresia 165
    and pulmonary stenosis 167
    reference ranges for 56, **224**
    rhythm strip 45, 62
    summary of 58
    in SVT 177
    and syncope 179
    and TAPVD 192
    technical settings of **44**
    and tetralogy of Fallot 188
    and tricuspid atresia 200
    and truncus arteriosus 201
    and VSD 205
    and VT 206, 208
    and WPW 209–10, **209**
    written reports of 44
echo assessment 60, 63, 194

echocardiogram
  and ALCAPA 67
  and aortic coarctation 95
  and aortic stenosis 70
  and ASD 76
  and bicuspid aortic valve 82
  and cardiac failure 86
  and cardiac output 21
  and cardiomyopathy 87, 89
  and DORV 101
  and duct-dependent
    circulation 102
  and Ebstein's anomaly 105
  fetal 110
  and hypertension 121
  and hypoplastic left heart
    123
  and IAA 130
  and Kawasaki disease 134
  and mitral regurgitation 138
  and mitral stenosis 139
  and myocarditis 144
  normal **60**
  and pericardial effusion **154**,
    155
  and pulmonary atresia 165
  and TAPVD 190, 192
  and tetralogy of Fallot 188
  and tricuspid atresia 200
  and truncus arteriosus 201
  unclear 62
  and VSD 206
  and VT 208
ECMO (extracorporeal
  membrane oxygenation) 106,
  107-8
  and Berlin Heart 81
  and cardiomyopathy 87
  and CPB 90
  and heart failure 85
  and PPHN 159
  in pre-transplant patients
    194
  and TAPVD 192
Edwards syndrome 101, 176,
  182, 203, 214
Ehlers–Danlos syndrome 137,
  176, 182
Eisenmenger syndrome 106–9,
  160, 204
ejection systolic murmur 70, 76,
  109, 140, 167, 189
Ellis–van Creveld syndrome 73
enalapril 27, 85
encephalopathy 32
enoximone 26
Enterococci 125
epistaxis 121
Epstein-Barr virus 144, 153
erythema marginatum 174
exercise testing 57, 61–2, 70,
  208
exercise tolerance, reduced 68,
  85, 138

extended matching questions
  (EMQs) 2–5
extremities, cold 28–9

Fabry disease 88–9
face, inspection of 37
failure to thrive 79, 85
familial Mediterranean fever
  153
fascicles 14
fatigue
  and aortic coarctation 95
  and aortic regurgitation 68
  and cardiac rejection 195
  and Eisenmenger syndrome
    109
  and infective endocarditis
    127
  and medications 29, 32
  and pulmonary hypertension
    161
  and pulmonary stenosis 167
FBC (full blood count)
  and cardiomyopathy 89
  and heart failure 85
fenestration 112
fetal cardiology 110–11
fever
  and infective endocarditis
    127
  and Kawasaki disease 133
  and myocarditis 143–5
  and pericarditis 157
FISH 165, 202
flecainide 23, 27, 32, 92, 210
fluconazole 30
fluid resuscitation 22, 23, 33,
  60
flushing 28, 30, 34–5
Fontan procedure 91, 100,
  111–12, **113**, 148–9, 199
foramen ovale
  fetal 16
  mixing at 192
  in newborns 13
  patent, *see* PFO
Friedreich's ataxia 88
frontal axis 45–7, **46–8**
fundoscopy 40, 121
furosemide 26, 32, 85

gallop rhythm 86, 103, 145, 195
gastroenteritis 134
Gaucher's disease 89
genetic screening 90, 208
GI (gastrointestinal)
  disturbances 29, 32, 34
glaucoma 28–9
Glenn shunt 91, 100, 105,
  111–12, 114–15, **114**
  bidirectional 147–8
glomerular disease 120
glycogen storage diseases 54,
  88–9

Goldenhar syndrome 176, 182
gout 32
great vessels **13**
  transposition of, *see* TGA
growth charts 40

haemodynamic compromise
  and cardioversion 92
  and pericardial effusion
    154–5
  and SVT 179
  and VT 208
Haemophilus 125
haemoptysis 109, 139, 161
hallucinations 29, 32
hands, inspection of 37
head injury 168, 215
headache
  and aortic coarctation 95
  and hypertension 121
  and infective endocarditis
    127
  and medications 28, 33–5
hearing loss
  and long QT 169–70
  sensorineural 169–70, 182–4
heart, structure of 11–14, **13**
heart block
  and adenosine 28
  complete (third-degree) **118**
  congenital 96, 110, 118
  first-degree 54, 116–17, **116**
  and medications 28, 31
  post operative 15, 119
  second-degree 31, 117–18,
    117
heart disease
  acquired 64–5, 173
  acyanotic 72
  congenital, *see* congenital
    heart disease
  cyanotic 158, 190, 198
  ischaemic 121
  structural 110, 119, 159, 207
heart-lung transplantation 161
heart murmur 139–40
  and aortic coarctation 95
  in aortic regurgitation 69
  and ASD 75–6
  and AVSD 75–6, 79
  and cardiomyopathy 90
  grading and timing of 39
  and myocarditis 145
  and rheumatic fever 175
heart rate
  calculating 45
  and cardiac cycle 18
  and cardiac output 21
  control of 23–4
  in exercise testing 62
  and LBBB 50
  medications increasing 28
  in newborns 16
  normal 23, **38**

heart rate (*continued*)
and QT interval 55, 168
reference ranges **24**
and SVT 178–9
heart sounds (HS)
in auscultation 38–9
and cardiac cycle **20**
fixed splitting of 76
muffled 155
and murmurs 127–8, **141**,
142
and TAPVD 192
and tetralogy of Fallot 189
and TGA 198
third 195
heaves 38
and aortic stenosis 70
and Eisenmenger syndrome
109
palpation of 11
and pulmonary hypertension
161
and TAPVD 192
hepatitis 134
hepatomegaly
and aortic coarctation 95
and AVSD 79
and duct-dependent
circulation 103
and heart failure 40, 86
and hypoplastic left heart
123
and pulmonary hypertension
161
HOCM (hypertrophic
obstructive cardiomyopathy)
69, 87–8, 90, 179, 217
Holt–Oram syndrome 73, 176,
182, 203
Holter monitor 61, 170
Hurler syndrome 89
hyperaldosteronism 120, 213
hyperglycaemia 29, 32
hyperkalaemia 34–5, 51, 53,
207–8, 215
hyperoxia test 97–8, 102
hypertension 119–20
following hypoxaemia 158
and medications 29–34
post-operative 94–5
pulmonary, *see* pulmonary
hypertension
secondary 119–20, 214
systemic 52, 120
and VACTERL association
185
young onset 94
hypertrophic cardiomyopathy
88, 180, 214
hypocalcaemia 130, 168, 181,
207, 215
hypoglycaemia 29, 207
hypokalaemia 30–1, 53–4, 116,
168, 207, 215

hypomagnesaemia 168, 207,
215
hyponatraemia 30, 35
hypoparathyroidism 181
hypoplastic left heart syndrome
(HLHS) 13, 122–3, **122**
antenatal detection of 111
and aortic coarctation 93
and bicuspid aortic valve 82
and BT shunt 83
and DILV 100
and duct-dependent
circulation 102
and Fontan procedure **112**
and mitral stenosis 138
and Rashkind procedure 171
repairing 146
and ventricular size 13
hypoplastic right heart
syndrome 115, 198
hypotension
acute 28, 33
and aortic coarctation 95
and cardiac rejection 195
and medications 29–30,
33–5
and pericardial effusion 155
postural 30, 32, 180, 214
hypothermia 24, 168, 215
hypothyroidism
and Down syndrome 181
and long QT 215
and medications 29
and pericardial effusion 154
and pericarditis 156
and T waves 53
hypovolaemia 97
hypoxaemia 157–8, 197
hypoxia
fetal 15
inotropic effect of 23
and PDA 150
and tetralogy of Fallot 187
in TGA 197
and VT 207
hypoxic seizures 180

IAA (interrupted aortic arch)
128–30, **129**
and aortic stenosis 69
and bicuspid aortic valve 82
and DiGeorge syndrome 181
and duct-dependent
circulation 102
and heart failure 214
and truncus arteriosus 201
ICD (implantable cardioverter
defibrillator) 87, 169, 208
immunosuppressants 194–5
indomethacin 152
infective endocarditis 124–7,
125
as acquired 65
and aortic regurgitation 67

and echocardiograms 61
and mitral regurgitation 137
and rheumatic fever 175
and tetralogy of Fallot 188
infundibular hypertrophy 187
innocent murmurs 127–8, 140,
218
inotropes 24, 85, 207
inotropic effects 22–3
inspection 36–7
intracranial bleeds 95, 121
intracranial pressure, raised
120, 213
ischaemia
myocardial 52, 84
peripheral 33
and ST segments 54, 70
and T waves 53
isomerism defects 119, 130–1
atrial 49, 59, 131
isoprenaline 119

Janeway lesions 126–7
Jatene procedure 71
Jervell and Lange–Nielsen
syndrome 169, 176, 183, 215
Jones criteria 174
jugular venous pressure (JVP)
38
raised 139, 155, 157, 161
juvenile idiopathic arthritis
(JIA) 156, 175

Kartagener's syndrome 131
Kawasaki disease 133–4
acquired 65
and aortic regurgitation 68
and cardiac catheterisation
62
and exercise testing 62
and mitral regurgitation 137
and Q waves 52
and rheumatic fever 175
and ST segments 54
Klippel–Feil sequence 176, 183
kyphoscoliosis 160, 183

LBBB (left bundle branch block)
48, 50, **51**, 144–5
left ventricle (LV)
dilated 90, 137
dominance of 52, 70, 165
double inlet, *see* DILV
position of 11, 13
in TGA 71–2
left ventricular hypertrophy
(LVH)
and aortic stenosis 70
and axis deviation 48
causes of 52
and dilated cardiomyopathy
88
and hypertension 120–1
and VSD 205

left ventricular volume overload 52
Leopard syndrome 88, 176, 183
lesions, duct-dependent 129, 152, 165, 217–18
lethargy 76, 121, 130, 138, 195
leukaemia 154, 175, 181
lidocaine 27, 32, 92, 208
lisinopril 27
lithium 32, 96, 105
liver function test (LFT) 30, 85, 134
long QT syndrome 168–9
 major causes of 215
 and medications 28–9
 and myocarditis 144
 and Romano–Ward syndrome 184
 and syncope 179–80
 and T waves 53, **170**
 and VT 206–8
losartan 27
lower respiratory tract infections 79, 192, 205
lung fields 216
LVAD (left ventricular assist device) **80**
LVOT (left ventricular outflow tract) obstruction 66, 69, 93, 158, 160, 172–3
Lyme disease 175

MAPCAs (major aortopulmonary collateral arteries) 164–5
Marfan syndrome 67–8, 137–8, 176, 183
meconium aspiration 97, 106, 157–8
meningitis, aseptic 134
metabolism, inborn errors of 88–9, 215
methaemoglobinaemia 33
methylprednisolone 195
methylxanthines 28
metoprolol 27
midline sternotomy scars 37, 90, 173
migraine 29, 73, 75, 180, 214
Miller's Pyramid **1**, 2
milrinone 26, 33, 85, 87
miscarriage, spontaneous 111
mitral atresia, and HLHS 122
mitral regurgitation 136–8, **136**
 and cardiac rejection 195
 murmur of 67, 86, 90
 and rheumatic fever 175
mitral stenosis 138–9
 and atrial hypertrophy 49
 and Eisenmenger syndrome 109
 and hypertrophic hearts 100
mitral valve apparatus **137**

mitral valve prolapse 127, 137, 183
mouth, inspection of 37
MRCPCH
 clinical examination circuit 6
 clinical examination mark scheme **7**
 examination structure 1–6
 standards for assessment **8–9**
MRI (magnetic resonance imaging) 57, 62–3, 95, 192
mucopolysaccharidoses 54, 88–9, 215
mumps 144, 153
Mustard procedure 142–3, **143**, 176, 198
myocardial depression 32, 197
myocardial infarction (MI)
 and ALCAPA 67
 and cardiomyopathy 215
 and medications 34
 medications for 29, 32
 and Q waves 51
 and ST segments 53
 and tetralogy of Fallot 187–8
myocarditis 143–5
 acquired 65
 and cardiomyopathy 215
 and heart block 116, 119
 investigations for 85
 and Kawasaki disease 134
 and pericardial effusion 153
 and PR interval 54, 215
 and rheumatic fever 175
 and T waves 53
 and VT 207
myocardium
 in ALCAPA 67
 and cardiac function 14, 22
myotonic dystrophy 88, 215

nadolol 169
necrotising enterocolitis 150
neonatal life support (NLS) 102
nephritic syndrome 34
nifedipine 27
nitric oxide 33–4, 149, 159, 161
nitrogen washout test 97, 197–8
Noonan syndrome 176, 183
 and ASD 73
 associated cardiac abnormalities 214
 and axis deviation 48
 and cardiomyopathy 88
 and PAPVD 193
 and pulmonary stenosis 166
noradrenaline 22, 26, 31, 33
Norwood procedure 146–9, **147**
 and BT shunt 83
 and cardiac catheterisation 62
 and CPB 91
 and DILV 100
 and Fontan procedure 111

and Glenn shunt 115
and hypoplastic left heart 122
nuchal translucency 110–11

obesity, and hypertension 121
organ damage
 and hypertension 120–1
 and hypoperfusion 85
Osler's nodes 37, 126–7
oxygen saturations 37, 62, 83, 102
oxygenation index 106

P wave
 and ASD 76
 assessment of **49–50**
 and Eisenmenger syndrome 109
 interpretation of 43
pacemakers
 and cardiomyopathy 87
 and heart block 118–19
 and long QT 169
 and MRI scans 63
 natural 14, 23
pain 23, 120, 155, 194, 213
pallor 36, 67, 85
palpation 11, 36–8, 40
palpitations
 and aortic regurgitation 68
 and ASD 76
 and Ebstein's anomaly 105
 in exercise testing 62
 and medications 28
 and mitral regurgitation 138
 and mitral stenosis 139
 and myocarditis 145
 and SVT 179
 and syncope 180
 and VT 207, 208
 and WPW 210
pancarditis 174–5
pancreatitis 32
pansystolic murmur 105, 138, 206
papillary muscles 43, 67, 136–7
PAPVD (partial anomalous pulmonary venous drainage) 12, 75, 192–3, **193**
parasympathetic supply 24
parenchymal disease 120
Parkinson's disease 175
Patau syndrome 101, 176, 184, 203
PDA (patent ductus arteriosus) 150–2
 definition of 16
 as acyanotic 65
 and aortic coarctation 93, 95
 and duct-dependent circulation 101–2
 and Eisenmenger syndrome 108

PDA (*continued*)
  ligation of 91
  and lung fields 216
  and Patau syndrome 184
  and pulmonary atresia 162,
   164
  and rubella 96
  and TAPVD 192
  and TGA 198
pedal oedema 86
percussion 36, 38
pericardial effusions 11, 59,
  152–5, **153–4**, 194–5
pericardial tamponade 38
pericarditis 155–7
  acquired 65
  and Kawasaki disease 134
  and pericardial effusion 153,
   155
  and rheumatic fever 175
  and ST segments 53
  susceptibility to 11
pericardium 11, 152, 155–6
permanent junctional
  reciprocating tachycardia 49
PFO (patent foramen ovale) 16,
  73–4, **74**, 163–5, 196–7
phaeochromocytoma 29, 31,
  120, 213
phenylketonuria 96
phosphodiesterase inhibitors
  26, 33
photographic material 4
PICU (Paediatric Intensive Care
  Unit) 21, 90, 106, 121
pleural effusion 86, 115, 195
Pneumococcus 153
pneumonia 115, 158
pneumonitis 29, 32
pneumothorax 58–9, 130, 183,
  217
polyarthritis 174–5
polycystic ovarian syndrome
  (PCOS) 34
polycythaemia 37, 97, 109
polysplenia syndrome 131
Pompe disease 51, 54, 88, 215
porphyria 30, 32, 35
potassium channel blockers 27
PPHN (persistent pulmonary
  hypertension of the newborn)
  157, 159
  aetiology of 160
  causes of 15
  and cyanosis 97
  and ECMO 106
  and medications 33
PR interval
  and ASD 76
  assessment of 54
  and AVSD 79
  and cardiac conduction 23
  and heart block 116–17
  interpretation of 23, 43

  long 105, 116, 183
  short 54, 209–10
praecordium 37, 140
  active 152
  dynamic 76, 79, 206
pregnancy, and medications
  29–30, 33, 35
propranolol 27, 169
prostacyclin 161
prostaglandin 34
  and aortic coarctation 94
  and aortic stenosis 69
  and cyanosis 98, 101
  and duct-dependent
   circulation 102
  and hypoplastic left heart
   122
  and IAA 129
  and pulmonary atresia 164
  and pulmonary stenosis 167
  and TGA 198
  and tricuspid atresia 199
  and truncus arteriosus 201
prostatic hypertrophy 29
prosthetic valves 124, 126
proteinuria 121
pulmonary artery (PA)
  band 91, 100–1, 161–2, **162**,
   199, 205
  branch stenosis 96, 185
  hypertension 63, 159–61
  pressure 107, 151, 158
pulmonary atresia 162–5,
  163–4
  and BT shunt 83
  and CXR 59
  as cyanotic 97
  and duct-dependent
   circulation 101
  and Rashkind procedure 171
  and VSD 203
pulmonary blood flow
  high 65
  reduced 66, 165, 187, 205,
   216
pulmonary circulation 12
pulmonary flow murmurs 128,
  192
pulmonary function,
  monitoring 62
pulmonary haemorrhage 150
pulmonary hypertension 161
  and ASD 73
  and atrial hypertrophy 49
  and blood pressure 121
  on ECG 76, 79
  and Eisenmenger syndrome
   106–8
  and lung fields 216
  and mitral regurgitation 137
  and mitral stenosis 138–9
  physiology of **159**
  and Rashkind procedure 171
  and syncope 180, 214

  and ventricular hypertrophy
   52
  and VSD 206
pulmonary oedema
  and aortic coarctation 95
  and cardiac rejection 195
  and cardiomyopathy 89
  and heart failure 86
  and medications 28
  and mitral regurgitation 138
pulmonary stenosis (PS) 165–7
  as acyanotic 66
  and chest X-ray 59
  critical 83, 102, 165, 167, 216
  and DORV 100–1
  and Klippel–Feil sequence
   183
  and Noonan syndrome 183,
   214
  peripheral 181
  and PPHN 158
  and Rastelli procedure 173
  and tetralogy of Fallot 186
  and TGA 72, 196
  and ventricular hypertrophy
   52
  and Williams syndrome 214
pulmonary vascular resistance
  in ALCAPA 67
  delayed fall in 158
  high 15, 65, 108, 157–8, 204
  measuring 62
  and medications 30
  in newborns 16
pulmonary vasodilation 28,
  149, 159
pulmonary veins, visualisation
  of 61
pulmonary venous congestion,
  and heart failure 86
pulmonary venous drainage; *see*
  also PAPVD; TAPVD
  and AVSD 77
  and isomerism 131
pulses 37–8
  absent 37, 82, 86, 95, 103,
   123
  bounding 152
  collapsing 69, 152
  in VT 207
pulsus paradoxus 155–7
Purkinje fibres 14, 43
pyrexia 34, 127–8, 195
pyuria 134

Q waves 51–2
QRS axis, *see* frontal axis
QRS complex
  assessment of 50–2
  and cardiac conduction 23
  and cardiac cycle 20
  and cardiac rejection 195
  and heart block 116, 118
  and heart rate 45

interpretation of 43
P wave hidden in 50
regularity of 45
in SVT 177
and VT 206, 208
QT interval
assessment of 55
in exercise testing 62
interpretation of 43, 168
prolonged, *see* long QT
syndrome
QTc (corrected QT value) 55,
130, 168–70

R waves, and ventricular
hypertrophy 52
radiofrequency ablation 178,
208, 210
rash 30, 133–4
Rashkind procedure 171, **172**,
198
Rastelli procedure 171, **172–3**,
198
RBBB (right branch bundle
block) 48, 50, **51**, 76, 79, 183
re-entry tachycardia 176–7
receptor sites 25–6, **26**
renal artery stenosis 120, 185,
213
renal impairment 30, 32–4, 121
renal perfusion 31
renal scarring 120, 213
renal vein thrombosis 120, 213
respiratory defects, congenital
97
respiratory distress
and AVSD 79
and cyanosis 97
and duct-dependent
circulation 103
and ECMO 106
and PPHN 157
and TAPVD 192
and truncus arteriosus 201
restrictive cardiomyopathy **89**,
180, 214
retinal haemorrhage 121
rheumatic fever 173–5
acquired 65
acute **174**
and aortic regurgitation 68
and heart block 116
and mitral regurgitation 137
and mitral stenosis 138
and pericardial effusion 153
and pericarditis 156
and PR interval 54
rheumatoid arthritis 118, 153,
156
rhythm, assessment of 45
rhythm strip 44–5, 49, 92, 206
rifampicin 30
right ventricle (RV)
dominance of 45, 52

double outlet, *see* DORV
in fetus 15
hypoplastic 112
and MRI 63
position of 11, 13
and sildenafil 34
right ventricular hypertrophy
(RVH)
and axis deviation 48
causes of 52
and chest X-ray 59
on ECG **52**
and heaves 38
and pulmonary hypertension
159–60
and T waves 53
and TAPVD 192
and tetralogy of Fallot 186–8
and TGA 197
rigors 125
Romano–Ward syndrome 176,
184, 215
Ross Procedure 70
Roth spots 126
RR interval 43, 45, 55
rubella 96, 151, 166
RVOT (right ventricular outflow
tract) obstruction 66, 173,
186, 188

salbutamol 24
SAN (sinoatrial node)
and heart rate 23
and isomerism 49, 131
and medications 28–9
role of 14
and syncope 180, 214
Sano modification 146–7
scars 36–7, 90
seizures
and cyanosis 97
and hypertension 121
and long QT syndrome 169
and syncope 179–80, 214
Senning procedure **143**, 198
sepsis 21, 85, 97, 158, 217
septic arthritis 134
septic shock 31, 33
septicaemia 157
Shone's Complex 138
shortness of breath
and aortic regurgitation 68
and aortic stenosis 70
and cardiac failure 85
and duct-dependent
circulation 102
and mitral regurgitation 138
and myocarditis 144
and TAPVD 192
sick sinus syndrome 28–9, 35,
180, 214
sildenafil 30, 33–4, 161
simvastatin 30
single ventricles 108, 111, 146

sinus arrhythmia 45
sinus rhythm
definition of 45
and arrhythmia 51
and AVSD 79
and tricuspid atresia 200
sinus tachycardia
and ALCAPA 67
and cardiac failure 86
and cardiac rejection 195
and CHD 95
and HLHS 123
and SVT **178**
and TAPVD 192
and VSD 205
sinus venosus ASD 73, 75–6, **76**
sinusitis, chronic 131
situs inversus 130–1
Sjögren's syndrome 118
sleep 24, 169
sodium channel blockers 27, 32
sotalol 27
spironolactone 27, 34–5, 85
splinter haemorrhages 37, 127
ST elevation 50, 53, 156
ST interval, interpretation of 43
ST segments 41–3, 53–4, **54**,
67, 130
Staphylococcus 125, 153
Starling's Law 21–2, **22–3**
sternotomy scars 90
steroids 120, 174, 194, 213
Still's murmur 127
stillbirth 111
Streptococcus 125, 153, 174
stress 24, 169
stroke 72–3, 121
subclavian artery 82–3, 94, 129,
146, 150
subclavian flap repair 94
sudden cardiac death
and ALCAPA 67
and cardiomyopathy 89
and Ebstein's anomaly 105
family history of 169–70,
179
and HCM 88
and heart transplant 194
high risk of 87, 169
and long QT 168
and Mustard procedure 143
and WPW 210
surfactant deficiency 97, 217
surgical procedures
non-bypass 91
palliative 194
SVC (superior vena cava), in
cardiac anatomy 12
SVT (supraventricular
tachycardia) 176–9, **177**
antenatal detection of 110
APLS algorithm for 178
and cardiac output 21
and cardioversion 92

SVT (*continued*)
  and medications 28, 31–2
  and QRS complex 51
  and sinus tachycardia **178**
  and WPW 209–10
'Swiss Cheese Defect' 204
syncope 179–80, 214
  and aortic stenosis 70
  and ECG 61
  and Eisenmenger syndrome
    109
  exercise-induced 62
  and long QT 168, 170
  and pulmonary hypertension
    161
  and Romano–Ward
    syndrome 184
  and SVT 179
  and VT 208
systemic arterial hypertension
  68
systemic lupus erythematosus
  (SLE)
  and aortic regurgitation 68
  and CHD 96
  and heart block 118
  and mitral regurgitation 137
  and pericardial effusion 153,
    155
  and pericarditis 156
  and pulmonary hypertension
    160
  and rheumatic fever 175
systolic murmur
  and aortic coarctation 95
  grading of 39
  intensity 139
  and PDA 152
  and TGA 197–8

T wave
  assessment of **53**
  interpretation of 43
  and long QT syndrome 170
tachyarrhythmias 28, 31, 35,
  209–10
tachycardia
  definition of 45, 70
  and aortic coarctation 95
  and AVSD 79
  and cardiac rejection 195
  and cardiomyopathy 215
  and duct-dependent
    circulation 103
  and heart failure 85
  and hypoplastic left heart
    123
  and IAA 130
  and medications 28, 31
  and mitral stenosis 139
  and myocarditis 145
  and P waves 49
  paroxysmal 209
  and pericardial effusion 155

  and pericarditis 157
  and rheumatic fever 175
  and TAPVD 192
  and TGA 198
  and truncus arteriosus 201
  and VT 206, 208
tachypnoea
  and aortic coarctation 95
  and cardiac failure 85
  and hypoplastic left heart
    123
  and pericardial effusion 155
  and TAPVD 192
  and TGA 198
  and truncus arteriosus 201
Takayasu disease 68
TAPVD (total anomalous
  pulmonary venous drainage)
  190–2, **190–1**
  and CXR 59
  as cyanotic 97
  and Eisenmenger syndrome
    108
  and heart structure 12
  and lung fields 216
TCPC (total cavopulmonary
  connection), *see* Fontan
  procedure
tetralogy of Fallot (ToF) 186–8,
  187, 214
  and BT shunt 83
  and cardiopulmonary bypass
    91
  and CHARGE association 181
  as cyanotic 97
  and duct-dependent
    circulation 101
  and Goldenhar syndrome
    182
  and heart block 119
  and lung fields 216
  and murmur 142
  and phenylketonuria 96
  prevalence of 195
  and pulmonary stenosis 166
  and QRS complex 50
  and VACTERL association
    185
  and ventricular hypertrophy
    52
  and VSD 203
  and VT 207
TGA (transposition of the great
  arteries) 195–8, **196**
  antenatal detection of 111
  and chest X-rays 59
  as cyanotic 97
  and diabetes 96
  and DORV 100
  and duct-dependent
    circulation 102
  and endocarditis 126
  and heart block 119
  and heart structure 14

  and IAA 129
  and MRI 63
  surgical correction of 71,
    142–3, 171
  and VSD 203
thiazides 26, 30
thrills 38–9
  and aortic stenosis 70
  and murmurs 127–8, 140
  and tetralogy of Fallot 189
  and VSD 204
thrombocytosis 33, 134
thromboembolic events 75, 81,
  112, 138
thrombus formation,
  intracardiac 61
thyrotoxicosis 29, 144
thyroxine 24
transient ischaemic attacks 121
Treacher–Collins syndrome
  176, 184
tricuspid atresia 198–200, **199**
  and axis deviation 48
  and BT shunt 83
  as cyanotic 97
  and diabetes 96
  and duct-dependent
    circulation 102
  and Fontan procedure 112
  and Glenn shunt **114**, 115
  and hypertrophic hearts 100
  and ventricular size 13
tricuspid regurgitation 49,
  104–5, 158, 160
tricuspid valve
  and Ebstein's anomaly 104–5
  position of 13
trisomy 13, *see* Patau syndrome
trisomy 18, *see* Edward
  syndrome
trisomy 21, *see* Down syndrome
truncus arteriosus 200–2, **200**,
  214
  as cyanotic 97
  and diabetes 96
  and DiGeorge syndrome 181
  and IAA 129
  and pulmonary hypertension
    160
tuberculosis 144, 153, 156
tuberous sclerosis 176, 184
Turner syndrome 93, 176, 184,
  193, 214

U wave, interpretation of 43
ultrasound, *see* echocardiogram
univentricular repair 62, 111
uraemia 154, 156
urinalysis 40, 121
urinary tract infections 120, 213
uveitis 134

VACTERL association 176, 185
vagus nerve 24, 29

Valsalva manoeuvre 178
vasculitis 68, 133
vasoconstriction 25–6, 28–31,
  97, 139
vasodilation 25, 30–1, 33
vegetations 124–5
velocardiofacial syndrome 129,
  164, 201
venous hum 128, 140
ventilation 87, 102, 194
ventricular assist device (VAD)
  80–1
ventricular ectopic beats 195,
  217
ventricular fibrillation (VF) 28,
  32, 168, 207–8, 210
ventricular hypertrophy 48,
  51–2, **52**, 59, 69, 95, 197
verapamil 27, 29, 35
vision, blurred 29, 34, 121
vomiting
  and Glenn shunt 115
  and medications 28–9, 31,
    33, 35
VSD (ventricular septal defect)
  203–6, **205**

definition of 13
as acyanotic 65
and alcohol 96
and aortic coarctation 93
and aortic stenosis 69
and chest X-ray 59
and cyanotic disease 66
and DiGeorge syndrome
  181
and DORV 100–1
and Eisenmenger syndrome
  108
and endocarditis 124
and Goldenhar syndrome
  182
and IAA 129–30
and lung fields 216
murmur of 101, 130, 142,
  165, 200
and PA bands 162
and pulmonary atresia **163**
and QRS complex 50, 52
and Rastelli procedure 173
and tetralogy of Fallot 186,
  188
and TGA 196–7

and Treacher–Collins
  syndrome 184
and tricuspid atresia 199
and truncus arteriosus 201
VT (ventricular tachycardia)
  206–8, **206**
  APLS algorithm for 207
  and cardioversion 92
  and exercise testing 62
  and medications 28, 32,
    35
  polymorphic 168, 180,
    214
  and QRS complex 51
  and syncope 180, 214

Wenckebach Block **117**
wheeze 86
Williams syndrome 69, 166,
  176, 185, 214
Wilms' tumour 120, 213
WPW (Wolff–Parkinson–White)
  syndrome **209–10**
  and cardiac anatomy 14
  and medications 28, 31–2
  and PR interval 54, 215

CPD with Radcliffe

You can now use a selection of our books to achieve CPD (Continuing Professional Development) points through directed reading.

We provide a free online form and downloadable certificate for your appraisal portfolio. Look for the CPD logo and register with us at: www.radcliffehealth.com/cpd

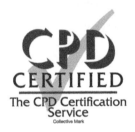

Printed and bound by CPI Group (UK) Ltd, Croydon, CR0 4YY

23/10/2024

01777678-0003